CUTTING THROUGH
THE SURFACE

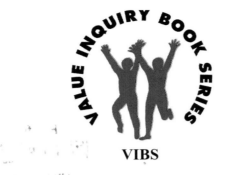

VIBS

Volume 211

Robert Ginsberg
Founding Editor

Leonidas Donskis
Executive Editor

Associate Editors

a volume in
Values in Bioethics
ViB
Matti Häyry and Tuija Takala, Editors

CUTTING THROUGH THE SURFACE

Philosophical Approaches to Bioethics

Edited by
Tuija Takala, Peter Herissone-Kelly,
and Søren Holm

Amsterdam - New York, NY 2009

Cover photo: Sibelius monument, Helsinki (© Morguefile)

Cover Design: Studio Pollmann

The paper on which this book is printed meets the requirements of "ISO 9706:1994, Information and documentation - Paper for documents - Requirements for permanence".

ISBN: 978-90-420-2739-8
E-Book ISBN: 978-90-420-2740-4
© Editions Rodopi B.V., Amsterdam - New York, NY 2009
Printed in the Netherlands

CONTENTS

FOREWORD

Philosophical bioethics is a challenging discipline. People who are concerned with practical matters often doubt the power of abstract theories to inform real-life decision making; while people with more academic outlooks tend to worry that bioethical topics are too close to our own lives to allow sufficient detachment. As a result, some criticize the discipline for being too theoretical and others criticize it for being too practical.

A feasible solution to this problem, adopted in many chapters of this book, is to focus on the clarity of concepts and the validity of arguments, and to present factual beliefs and moral convictions as tentative or hypothetical elements of ethical reasoning. This choice allows philosophers to work with the logical tools that they are trained to employ, *and* to provide enlightened decision makers with knowledge of the ways in which normative views have been and can be defended.

Another solution, also adopted in some chapters of this book, is to sketch full normative cases for or against particular policies or courses of action. This approach is preferred by public authorities and funding institutions due to its promise to deliver direct guidance. The soundness of the conclusions depends, of course, on the truth of the premises that have been used in the arguments; and as the truth of moral convictions is seldom a straightforward matter, the wisdom of following the guidance without further consultation and debate remains in most instances doubtful.

In this exquisite collection of new essays, some of my best friends write, in a celebratory mood and with their usual skill and flair, about my favorite issues in philosophical bioethics: methods, theories, principles, and responsibility. In many cases, our discussions on these themes have been ongoing for years—a fact evidenced by the number of references to our past exchanges. The topics are universal, and their treatment here has personal appeal to me partly because through the eyes of my friends I can see trends not only in my own work but in bioethics more generally.

Since bioethics comprises both practical regulation and theoretical studies, the approaches chosen by ethicists in different spheres are, justifiably, diverse. And since theoretical studies can be conducted in many ways—empirically, conceptually, historically, and so on—the methods selected by scholars are also, legitimately, many and varied. One of the greatest advances in the field of bioethics during the last few decades is that at least most academics have recognized these variations and learned to live with them without unnecessary antagonism.

Philosophers who are primarily interested in the intricacies of human thinking can use studies in bioethics to drive the development of their moral theories. (If the authors in this volume are correct, my thinking has during the last twenty years moved from a humane, positive mixture of liberalism and consequentialism to a grimmer, negative version of "Schopenhauerian utilitarianism"—which I did not know existed but which sounds intriguing.) As for applying moral theories to practice, however, the difficulty of incompatible normative premises looms large. To illustrate, consider the following three questions: "Why should I value dignity?" "Why should I value happiness?" "Why should I value tradition?" In conflict situations, responses to these vary from "I should not" to "Because it defines me as a person," with little understanding between people who answer the questions differently. Since the concepts of dignity, happiness, and tradition mark, however, the main strands in contemporary normative philosophical bioethics, it is unlikely that everyone will agree on practical conclusions reached by champions of just one fundamental notion.

People with more practical aims in mind have tried to bypass this problem by introducing a plethora of theoretically less demanding principles, agreeable to most and applicable to the bioethical issues that we face. This has led to the invention of the ethics of autonomy, beneficence, justice, care, trust, precaution, solidarity, vulnerability, and many others. As long as everyone remembers that all these words—like dignity, happiness, and tradition—have several meanings, their use in bioethical discussions is an unmixed blessing. New terms draw attention to new dimensions in ethical dilemmas and have a great potential of facilitating understanding. More caution is needed with normative results that are based on one particular principle or set of principles, interpreted in a way that excludes all other readings.

A theme explored in many chapters of this book is reproductive responsibility. Five years ago I published a short provocation arguing that *if* a certain popular view of rationality is correct and *if* a certain moral stance is tenable *then* it is irrational and immoral to have children. My commentators show conclusively that the positions on rationality and morality that I used are not universally accepted and that there are alternative outlooks according to which it is usually alright to make babies. While this reaction is unsurprising and perfectly compatible with my conditional thesis, the exciting detail here is to see how difficult it is to justify, by philosophical arguments, a simple everyday choice like the decision to have children.

My heartfelt thanks are due to the authors and editors of this wonderful collection of essays. I hope that others will enjoy reading it as much as I did.

Matti Häyry
Helsinki, July 2009

PREFACE

This is a book to celebrate Professor Matti Häyry's 50th birthday, on 20 September 2006. In August the same year the *European Society for Philosophy of Medicine and Health Care* held its annual conference in Helsinki and in that conference a Special Session was organized around the book. We wish to thank the Society and the local organizers for that opportunity, and the presenters and participants for their contributions. Those on the podium in Helsinki were: Timo Airaksinen, Gardar Árnason, Vilhjálmur Árnason, Rebecca Bennett, Anthony Mark Cutter, Heta Gylling, Matti Häyry, Sirkku Hellsten, Søren Holm, Harry Lesser, Pekka Louhiala, Rosamond Rhodes, Floora Ruokonen, Niall Scott, Margit Sutrop, Tuija Takala, and Simo Vehmas.

During the years it has taken to prepare this collection, we have received support from the following sources:

- Centre for Social Ethics and Policy, University of Manchester, UK
- Department of Social and Moral Philosophy, University of Helsinki, Finland
- European Society for Philosophy of Medicine and Health Care
- *NeuroSCAN (Neuroscience and Norms)*, a project funded by the Academy of Finland (SA 1124638)
- *Methods in Philosophical Bioethics* funded by the Academy of Finland (SA 131030)

The editors of this book acknowledge this support with gratitude.

Tuija Takala, Peter Herissone-Kelly, and Søren Holm
August 2009, Kirkkonummi, Finland; Preston and Cardiff, UK

Introduction

BIOETHICS:
WHAT LIES UNDER THE SURFACE?

Tuija Takala, Peter Herissone-Kelly, and Søren Holm

And they'll tell you black is really white
The moon is just the sun at night
And when you walk in golden halls
You get to keep the gold that falls
Its Heaven and Hell …
Oh well[1]

In 2003 Rodopi published a book edited by Matti Häyry and Tuija Takala titled *Scratching the Surface of Bioethics*. In the current volume, the aim is to dig deeper and to understand more about the elusive discipline called bioethics. Obviously bioethics is not only an academic field of study—or rather a cluster of academic disciplines—but also covers a number of practices from clinical bed-side bioethics to the work of regulative and legislative committees. The latter are not, however, the topic of this book. While the theoretical and practical sides of bioethics can and should learn from each other, the academic work has its own strict requirements concerning coherence, conceptual clarity, and validity of arguments that should not bend to accommodate practical concerns. Similarly, the nuances of practical problems should not be forgotten in attempts to use theories to solve questions in practical settings. This book is about the academic side of bioethics and more specifically about philosophical bioethics. While some of the papers study the interplay of the different approaches, the methods are those of philosophical bioethics.

Sometimes philosophical bioethics seems to be mere rhetoric, and indeed a skilled philosopher can twist and turn concepts, words, and arguments to justify almost any normative statement. However, one of the aims of this book is to show that bioethics should and can be more. In its 23 chapters bioethical theories, concepts, methods, values, principles, and norms are studied with adherence to the requirements of the discipline, yet with an understanding that the issues discussed are not pure abstractions, but refer to the often very serious issues dealt with by actual people in the real world.

1. What Is Bioethics?

The first three chapters deal with the question "What is bioethics and where should it be going?" In the opening chapter Sirkku Hellsten studies the very name of the field and its various usages. She suggests that much of the confusion in bioethics is caused by lack of common understanding of what the word "bioethics" means. In the article she explicates and explains the different meanings and roles given to "bioethics." In conclusion she envisages a future where the different approaches to bioethics can complement one another, but wishes to reserve a special place for philosophy because of the importance given to reflection and critical analysis in that field of study.

In his contribution, Sven Ove Hansson presents us with a new approach to ethics. He shows how the traditional distinction between moral philosophy and applied ethics in its various forms fails to respond to the need to create ethics that is relevant to the constantly changing social and natural environment.

In chapter three Harry Lesser takes a closer look at the theories of liberalism and utilitarianism with a view to discovering whether they can be combined to tackle bioethical problems. His suggestion for a way forward is a partnership model rising from a Millian type of liberal utilitarianism that could replace the old paternalistic attitudes without collapsing into pure consumerism.

2. How to Do Bioethics?

Chapters four to seven deal with ways of doing bioethics. The chapters by Veikko Launis and Juha Räikkä look at methodological issues, while Pekka Louhiala and Leila Toiviainen approach bioethics from the viewpoints of a medical doctor and a nurse, respectively.

The principlist approach to bioethics divides philosophers; some believe that it can solve all bioethical problems whilst others think that it creates more problems than it solves. In his paper, Veikko Launis offers a modest defense of the approach by showing how two of the main objections against principlism fail to prove the approach to be theoretically inadequate. Contrary to many critics, he finds the "lightness" of the principles quite bearable. In chapter five, Juha Räikkä examines the method of "wide reflective equilibrium." While he recognizes the strengths of the method he also claims that one's arguments are not made better by knowledge of methodological issues.

In his contribution, Pekka Louhiala studies the role of philosophers in medical ethics. He argues that both philosophers and medical doctors have a role in medical ethics and that they should acknowledge each others' value. In the following chapter Leila Toiviainen calls for recognition for nursing ethics.

She sees the nurse's position as unique within the field of health care and holds that bioethics needs more input from nursing.

3. Dignity, Precaution, and Solidarity

The contributors of part three of the book have been, at least partly, prompted to write their contributions by Matti Häyry's work on the concepts of dignity, precaution, and solidarity.[2] The part opens with an analysis of the concept of dignity by Simon Woods. In his chapter Woods sets out to defend the concept's usefulness in bioethics against some well-known claims to the contrary. Woods grants that there is some vagueness to the concept, but he holds that there is also significant moral substance to it that cannot be captured by alternative notions. In the following chapter Niall Scott continues on the same theme, by adding the notions of autonomy and freedom into the picture. He defends a Kantian notion of autonomy that upholds a person's dignity and can sometimes limit that person's freedom. Restricting someone's freedom is not, however, according to him an ethical but a practical question.

Michael Parker and Paolo Vineis turn our attention to the principle of precaution. They show how the current versions of the principle rest upon contestable claims, but continue their scrutiny by showing how, properly understood, the principle of precaution can be a valuable tool for assessing the acceptability of science and technology.

Chapters eleven and twelve have in common the ideas of solidarity and justice. In his contribution, Vilhjálmur Árnason studies Nordic healthcare systems and their struggle to justify prioritization. He argues that the Rawlsian notion of justice can, both as a procedural notion and as a critical idea, help the Nordic states maintain the solidarity of the systems.

Søren Holm discusses the problem of how to justify care for the elderly within a liberal framework. In the course of his chapter he shows how truly liberal justifications for the current welfare system are hard to come by and that also the cosmopolitan, liberal academic needs to rely on illiberal state enforced beneficence and, though he does not use the word, solidarity, to help him in old age.

4. Tests and Experiments

The chapters in part four of the book are interested in the notion of eradicating disease. In chapter thirteen, Margaret Battin and her colleagues study the ethical acceptability of large-scale rapid testing for infectious disease. They argue that the possibility of ridding ourselves of (many) infectious diseases is so beneficial that even a "decade of infectious-disease inconvenience" (minor infringements on liberty, privacy, and even justice) should be accepted.

John Harris looks at the ethics of animal testing through a report by the Nuffield Council in the United Kingdom. In his analysis he highlights various inconsistencies in the report and argues that the main issue that needs to be solved to settle the question of whether using (some/all) animals in research is justified is their moral status.

The last chapter of the part is by Rosamond Rhodes and tackles the issue of using human beings as research subjects. Rhodes argues that scientific research should be seen as a collaborative project in which researchers and research subjects have a shared interest in the advancement of medical sciences.

5. Rationality, Morality, and Reproduction

In response to the increased possibilities of choosing the kind of children we wish to have, bioethics needed to say something about whether making such choices is at all justified, and if it is, under what circumstances. Various arguments have been put forward to show the moral limits of such practices. In 2004 Matti Häyry published two articles in which he took some of these arguments to their logical conclusions and showed how, with certain presuppositions, human reproduction is not only irrational but also immoral.[3] The authors of this part have been, at least partly, provoked to write their contributions by these articles.

In chapter sixteen Floora Ruokonen and Simo Vehmas look at parental responsibility generally and study two assentist positions regarding parenthood in more detail. Their analysis shows that rights and duties might not be the most fitting tools for examining parental responsibility and suggests that a more virtue-oriented approach could facilitate the work.

All the other contributors to this section comment directly on Häyry's writing on the irrationality and immorality of reproduction. Frank J. Leavitt analyzes Häyry's notion of suffering and argues that it fails to understand full human existence of which suffering is a part. Richard Ashcroft puts Häyry's arguments in the context of his previous work and shows that there are some inconsistencies. In terms of the rationality of reproduction, Ashcroft argues that rationality is not necessarily the most appropriate measure of the acceptability of the reasons given for reproduction. Rebecca Bennett accepts that reproduction could well be irrational, but that does not, she maintains, render the activity immoral. In the course of her analysis, she shows how there could actually be more suffering in the world if reproduction were drastically limited. Tom Buller points out that reproduction is not exactly the lottery that Häyry seems to make it out to be; he would rather call it gambling. And in gambling, we can play the odds and thus, in reproduction too, we can shorten the odds in favor of our children.

6. Philosophical Responses to Enhancements

In chapter twenty-one Lisa Bortolotti continues on the theme of reproduction, but takes it one step further and argues that there are moral reasons for cognitively enhancing our children if and when this becomes safe and possible. In the paper she considers the main arguments against the view, but shows how these either confuse issues or are not about moral matters *per se*.

Heta Gylling discusses the topic of cosmetic surgery for aesthetic reasons. In her analysis she shows how many of the reasons supplied for our enhancing our appearance are suspect. She does not, however, condemn the practice as such, but sees the role of doctors (as professionals) especially ethically problematic.

The book ends with Timo Airaksinen's futuristic discussion of cyborgs. In his chapter he studies two types of cyborg theory and the possibility of new life forms. If the transhumanists are right in their predictions, it is in these kinds of discussions that the future of bioethics lies.

NOTES

1. Ronnie James Dio, lyrics, "Heaven and Hell" from the album *Heaven and Hell* by Black Sabbath (Vertigo, 1980).

2. *E.g.*, Matti Häyry, "European Values in Bioethics: Why, What, and How to be Used?" *Theoretical Medicine and Bioethics* 24 (2003), pp. 199–214; Matti Häyry, "Another Look at Dignity," *Cambridge Quarterly of Healthcare Ethics*, 13 (2004), pp. 7–14; Matti Häyry, "Precaution and Solidarity," *Cambridge Quarterly of Healthcare Ethics*, 15 (2005), pp. 199–205; Matti Häyry, "The Tension Between Self-Governance and Absolute Inner Worth in Kant's Moral Philosophy," *Journal of Medical Ethics*, 31 (2005), pp. 645–647.

3. Matti Häyry, "If You Must Make Babies, Then at Least Make the Best Babies You Can?" *Human Fertility*, 7 (2004), pp. 105–112; Matti Häyry, "A Rational Cure for Pre-Reproductive Stress Syndrome," *Journal of Medical Ethics*, 30 (2004), pp. 377–378; see also Matti Häyry, "The Rational Cure for Pre-Reproductive Stress Syndrome Revisited," *Journal of Medical Ethics*, 31 (2005), pp. 606–607; Matti Häyry, "An Analysis of Some Arguments For and Against Human Reproduction," *Arguments and Analysis in Bioethics*, eds. Matti Häyry, Tuija Takala, Peter Herissone-Kelly, and Gardar Árnason (Amsterdam and New York: Rodopi, 2009), pp. 167–175.

Part One

WHAT IS BIOETHICS AND
WHERE SHOULD IT BE GOING?

One

WHY "DEFINITIONS" MATTER
IN DEFINING BIOETHICS?

Sirkku K. Hellsten

1. Introduction

In this chapter I shall discuss how the definition of "bioethics" affects the practice and use of bioethical research today. As an academic field of study, bioethics covers a multiplicity of disciplines and a diversity of professional practices. It also encompasses a wealth of ethical views and belief systems. Depending on whether bioethics is studied or practiced by people working as heath care practitioners and medical researchers, or as philosophers, lawyers, theologians, and policy-makers, ideas on what is meant by "bioethics" vary greatly, as does understanding of the main concepts of bioethics.

There is no comprehensively shared understanding of what bioethics really is even among those who are one way or another involved in the discipline. Further there is no clear agreement on who "does" or "practices" bioethics, or indeed who should do or practice it. "Bioethicists" themselves also have different ideas on what it is that they actually do—or are supposed to do. There are debates concerning whether bioethics is—or should be—descriptive or prescriptive, what methodology is to be used in bioethical inquiry, and about what the goals of "bioethics" are.

This diversity of views and approaches to bioethics has led to a situation in which discussions on bioethical topics easily lose their focus, and turn into non-argumentative accounts of diverse views on different ethical questions. "Bioethics" as an academic discipline has gradually lost some of its earlier reflective edge. It now has a tendency to fall into epistemological and ethical relativism and uncritically support all possible approaches to the issues with which it deals. It no longer matters whether different views are validly argued for or not. Whether they rely on an analytical, empirical, or intuitive method of verification, they are all considered "equally valuable" and thus, "equally right." This chapter argues that if we cannot define what "bioethics" is all about in the first place, we cannot expect to have clear arguments that one or another form of bioethics is normatively more plausible than all others, or even logically more coherent. Thus, I suggest, if we want to make bioethics research "meaningful" again, we need to return to more analytical philosophical reflection on the issues of definitions, arguments, and logic.

2. Definitions and Ethics

Clear definitions are central to any philosophical analysis and argumentation, naturally including those in ethics. Particularly such concepts as life, death, health, well-being, human dignity, as well as justice, fairness, and equality are the starting points of reflective inquiry in ethics. However, during recent years it appears that conceptual analysis has become less popular in bioethical research, while the very concept of "bioethics" has simultaneously become more blurred and ambiguous, and its point of reference more uncertain.

Over the years philosophers have held various conflicting views about the purpose of definitions as such. For Plato, for instance, definitions were intended to explicate the meaning of certain eternal essences or forms, such as justice, piety, and virtue. For most philosophers and logicians today, however, definitions are intended exclusively to explicate the main meaning of words. Definitions are central to any valid and sound ethical argumentation that helps us to see the different sides of the issues at hand, and to find a common language for dialogue that involves both facts and values.[1]

Simply put, definitions are *summary statements* about the referents of our concepts. A good definition helps us to keep our intellectual filing system in order by giving us a summary of what is in each folder of the concepts we use. To define a word is to state the rules or conditions for using the word; to explain how the word is actually used or is going to be used.[2]

In order for us to manage our mental filing systems we need some basic rules for formulating good definitions. Particularly when engaging in ethical argumentation we need to be sure that the concepts we use are not defined too widely or too narrowly, and that they do not confuse the issues under discussion. For example, defining "human being" as "two legged animal" is too broad a definition, since it would also include birds. On the other hand a too narrow definition for "human being" is "religious animal," since this would exclude, for instance, atheists from the class of human beings. A good definition should state the essential attributes of the concept's referents. It should also avoid circular reasoning, vagueness, obscurity, and metaphor. For instance defining "death" as a "cessation of participation in finitude" is more difficult to grasp and agree on than "loss of life."

Particularly in relation to ethical argumentation, it is important not to include strong value judgments in definitions. We need to remember that definitions can also be used as means of persuasion when they engender a favorable or unfavorable attitude toward what is denoted by the definiendum. This purpose is accomplished by assigning an emotionally charged or value-laden meaning to a word, while making it appear that the word really has (or ought to have) that meaning in the language in which it is used. For example, "abortion" can be defined as "a ruthless murdering of an innocent human being," or as "a safe and established surgical procedure whereby a woman is relieved of an unwanted burden," or as "a medical termination of pregnancy."[3]

3. Defining Bioethics for a Particular Purpose?

Paying attention to definitions helps us to understand what we are talking about, and what we are agreeing or disagreeing on. Definitions are particularly important in bioethics, since the topics of reflection are complex and the relationship between facts and values is not always clear. It should also be recognized that sometimes definitions include some functional aspects of the concepts, and so present a certain inherent purpose.

The concept of "bioethics" itself particularly appears to have been defined in various different ways depending on what is seen as the ultimate purpose of the study, or what it is to be used for. The meaning of "bioethics" has also shifted depending on the context, occasion of use, cultural and belief setting, and the task at hand. For instance, at the inaugural Congress of the International Association of Bioethics in Amsterdam in 1992, the term "bioethics" needed to be defined and accepted for the Constitution of the Associations. In the invitation letter to the interested parties Peter Singer defined bioethics as, "the study of the ethical issues raised in health care and in the biological sciences," including, "the study of social, legal, and economic issues related to these ethical issues."[4]

This definition was followed by an enumeration of the Objectives of the Association such as to facilitate contacts, to organize international conferences, to encourage the development of research and teaching, and to uphold the values of free discussion in bioethics. This is a descriptive definition of bioethics. A prescriptive definition would be, for example, one that states that "the objective of bioethics is to consider how to maintain respect for human dignity and protect individuals in light of our expanding knowledge of the life sciences and their applications (for example, euthanasia, organ donation, cloning, embryo research)."[5]

The wide interest in bioethics has drawn it away from a narrower construal, philosophical bioethics, that (although it may have drawn from the other disciplines) is itself an area of philosophical inquiry. If we look up the word "bioethics" in philosophical dictionaries, teaching curricula, research papers, and bioethics associations' web-pages we can find various other definitions.

"Bioethics" has been defined for example as (emphasis mine):

– the *study of* the ethical, social, legal, philosophical and other related issues arising in the biological sciences and in health care.

— the *ethics of* biological research and the development and application of biotechnology, both within and beyond the human sphere.
– *ethics as applied to health care.*

The term "bioethics" was invented in 1970 by Van Rensselaer Potter, an oncology research scientist with a wide interest in biology and human values. Around the same time it was used by a Dutch physiologist and obstetrician Andre Hellegers, who referred with "bioethics" to a new discipline that combines "biological knowledge with the knowledge of human value system" and which would therefore build a bridge between the sciences and humanities; *help humanity to survive and sustain and improve the civilized world.*

— the word bioethics stems from two Greek words; "bios," which means life, and "ethikos," which means ethics or mores. Thus, the *study of bioethics unites multiple fields*: medical treatment, mores, politics, finance, and philosophy in holistic situations, and also considers issues about *public policies.*
— the *study of ethical issues arising in the practice of the biological disciplines.* These include medicine, nursing, and other health care professions, including veterinary medicine, and medical and other biological or life sciences.
– bioethics *concerns the relationships between biology, medicine, cybernetics, politics, law, ethics, philosophy, and theology.*[6]

While the above-mentioned definitions have a lot in common, they also have their differences, particularly in the focus they take. Disagreement also exists about the proper scope for the application of ethical evaluation to questions involving biology and the medical sciences. Some bioethicists would *narrow* the scope of such evaluation to include only the morality of medical treatments or technological innovations, and focus on the ethical aspects of medical practice, as well as the use and application of medical technology and medicine in general in a society. Other bioethicists would *broaden* the scope of ethical evaluation to include the morality of all actions that might help or harm organisms capable of feeling fear and pain. In its broadest sense, bioethics appears to cover almost all aspects of ethics, since ethics must be related to issues that involve human life, death, and suffering, as well as environmental values and the moral status of animals. In general, all definitions of "bioethics" make mention of value-related studies in bio- and life sciences. Most definitions agree that bioethics involves philosophy, but they hardly claim it to be philosophical study—or even an application of philosophical ethics. None of the above definitions restricts the methodology to be used to philosophical analysis. Instead, they focus on the topics of bioethics: ethical, legal, philosophical (and so on) *issues* or *questions* involved in the (bio)sciences.

4. Which Bioethics, Whose Ethical Inquiry?

Bioethical research includes a variety of academic disciplines such as moral philosophy, moral theology, law, economics, psychology, sociology, anthropology, and history, as well as biology and medicine. It also engages relevant professionals and practitioners such as doctors, nurses, and life scientists, along with their patients and research subjects. In addition, it one way or another includes the public in general, both as individuals, and as members of various interest groups. Political representatives also increasingly take a distinct interest in bioethics issues, as do the media.

In order to gain some clarity about the definition of "bioethics," there have been attempts further to specialize the different approaches to the discipline. This has led to trends in bioethical inquiries, which focus on a particular set of questions within the wider field of bioethics. However, this differentiation has not brought clarity to the definition of bioethics *per se*; instead, it has widened the scope of the discipline further, while simultaneously limiting the questions to be discussed from a particular perspective or normative stance within one or another strand of "bioethics." Here I am referring to approaches to bioethical questions such as feminist bioethics, global bioethics, theological bioethics, or non-Western bioethics. Feminist bioethics pays particular attention to women's rights and gender disparities in relation to social injustices, while global bioethics focuses on global injustices in medicine, medical technology, pharmaceutical markets, property rights, human rights, and environmental science, as well as on cultural differences in the context of bioethics. Theological bioethics for its part focuses on religious responses and considerations to the ethical issues related to medicine, new technology, and the environment. Non-Western bioethics brings in different cultural approaches that mainly discuss bioethics in a comparative context (Japanese, Chinese, Latin American, African, and so on). New fields of bioethics inquiry have also emerged, such as "Health and Human Rights," which combines ethical inquiry with medical law and international law.

The last area is particularly difficult, since there already exists a muddle between law and ethics, and the particular connection between bioethics and human rights as a field of study blurs the difference between legal and moral aspects of ethical issues even further. In a similar vein, mixing applied ethics with cultural anthropology or sociology tends to confuse the normative and descriptive aspects of ethical investigations. Studies in social sciences are usually aimed at describing what the case is or how things are, and while anthropologists or sociologists can tell us what members of particular communities think about certain practices, this should not be confused with how things should, morally, be. Sometimes, however, these descriptions are understood as prescriptions. The result is that the normative and descriptive elements of ethical inquiry become hopelessly tangled together.[7]

Philosophical ethics for its part should involve advanced examination of arguments concerning what ought or ought not to be done, morally speaking, or what is morally right or wrong. In relation to bioethics, the question has been whether it should remain as an abstract, theoretical pursuit, describing and exploring the moral construction that society is building around life sciences, or whether it should be more pragmatic, offering moral guidance to all who are affected by the rapid development of the sciences, including medicine. Is bioethics "ethics as usual" or is it normative ethical inquiry that promises real world solutions to real world problems?

The practitioners and scientists tend to prefer the latter account, since they need clear guidelines as how to do research, how to deal with new technologies, and how to apply them in practice, in relation to human beings animals, and the environment—so long as these guidelines are practical and do not frustrate the development of science. Religious groups often heavily oppose this approach; expressing fears that bioethics will turn into a new "biopolitics," that will allow human beings/scientists to do experiments that are "unnatural" from religious points of view. Instead the religious bioethicists would like to see a strictly normative, deontological approach that prevents science from taking the role of God in both an ethical and an evolutionary sense.[8]

5. "Ought" from "Is"?

While bioethics is, academically speaking, still a sub-field of philosophical ethics, when practiced today—as embedded in formal governmental regulations, state laws, and a myriad of other documents, committees, guidelines, and guidebooks—it often deliberately or inadvertently takes a normative stance toward various issues related to the development of the sciences. Neutral ethics is difficult even philosophically speaking, since ethical inquiry in general studies what is right and wrong, good or bad. However, when non-philosophers who are either practitioners or come from other disciplines want to engage in bioethics, the distinction between normative and descriptive often becomes even more vague. As noted earlier, when disciplines are mixed, sometimes facts are presented as values, and vice versa. For example: "Apples have many vitamins. Thus, it is right to eat apples every day" may turn from a merely practical recommendation to an ethical one. Similarly, we could state that because many embryos are destroyed in stem cell research, and human material wasted in the process, stem cell research is bad and wrong. However, to make the normative claim we should be able to show what, if anything, is intrinsically valuable about apples or human material. The tendency to draw an "ought" from an "is" (known as the naturalistic fallacy) is even stronger in bioethics than it is in traditional ethical inquiry. Scientific explanations are easily confused with reflective analytical argumentation—descriptive and normative elements of either explanations or arguments are mixed together and generalizations on conclusions are swiftly drawn. Even such early analytical approaches as that taken by Peter Singer in relation to the moral status of "personhood" have been interpreted by various religious or disability activist groups as normative attempts to degrade the value of the lives of those who are, theoretically speaking, "less than perfectly rational and capable."

It should be kept in mind that natural sciences or the social sciences cannot directly mediate ethical claims. A false sense of superiority is often assumed by those bioethicists who assert that their conclusions are inconvertible because they are "scientific." Closer examination of these claims reveals considerable confusion about the boundaries between science and belief. Confusion is often evident in discussions about the beginning and the end of human life. Here, for example, science may establish that a genetically distinct human individual comes into existence at fertilization. Science, and strictly speaking natural sciences, however, cannot establish whether this being is a human person or what are the ethically acceptable characteristics or attributes of moral agency. These are philosophical questions, and science is not competent to decide philosophical questions. Similarly, science cannot determine what moral obligations are called forth by the existence of a human individual. Questions about human values are not scientific in nature, and neither can science determine our moral obligations. Science, however, can produce important factual data that philosophical ethicists can incorporate into their deliberations. Discussing values, norms, and moral principles requires the sort of critical reflection and sound argumentation that is characteristic of philosophical research.[9]

At the same time, theological bioethics may have a point in fearing that secular ethics attempts to base moral guidelines on reason or logic without giving due consideration to the "deeper" sources of ethics. Secular bioethics may claim to offer a "neutral" ethical vision, because the approach has its moral foundation in secular principles rather than in religious beliefs. However, it is an error to assume that what is called secular is unencumbered by metaphysical or moral presuppositions. In reality all ethical systems—secular or religious—make use of certain assumptions about human values, and about what is right and wrong, and these assumptions are dependent on the overall context and values of the society in which the arguments are constructed. Scientific research is to improve human condition and well-being.

To discuss the ethics of euthanasia, for example, is to ask whether euthanasia is "right" or "wrong." This question cannot be decided without defining "right" or "wrong," or dismissing the very concepts as irrelevant or erroneous. As Murphy notes, in this sense secularists are believers too: they believe that human dignity exists, that human life is worthy of respect, and so on. These are principles that can be accepted on faith and are not a matter of scientific fact. Secular ethicists might, however, try to build a consistent argumentative defense of the principles in which they believe. They might be believers in liberalism, utilitarianism, or Kantian deontology, and believe in the supremacy of one particular political or ethical framework over the others. Secular bioethics may also ignore the role of truly reflective philosophical analysis.[10]

6. Bioethics or Biopolitics?

The diversity in approaches, methodology, and understanding of the purpose of bioethics has gradually led to a situation in which bioethics no longer aims for, or respects, philosophical argumentation and rigor, and in which it can always be redefined according to the purpose that is given to it, depending on the context in which it is used. Those who are "experts" in bioethics (many after quite a brief or narrow education in the field) can then easily be used by the policy makers, politicians, or by whomever who has more practical interests in bioethical matters.

Since bioethics involves many public policy questions, there is always a danger that the definition itself will become politicized, and is then used to mobilize political constituencies and political agendas. Some see "bioethics" as a utilitarian monster which aims to destroy the value of life, and to undermine human dignity and individual rights. For others "bioethics" is an attempt to bring wisdom and values to bio- and life sciences in a way that helps us to understand better the complexities of modern life, the latest technology, and scientific discovery. The purpose and scope of bioethics can easily be defined according to the interests of the organizations in question (for instance, government bodies, private and public health care agencies, international policy makers, religious organizations, and various activist groups). Different interest groups use the "experts" that best fit their cause, and are most likely to come up with conclusions favorable to the views of their organizations. The danger in this is that bioethics leads into biopolitics, as Michel Foucault has pointed out. When concepts like "normality," "health," and "illness" are defined in a manner that, either deliberately or inadvertently, provides ideals with in-built value judgments about what is desirable in a society, the result is inequality and stigmatization of those who do not meet the criteria set for "(desirable) human life." When an ethical "ought" is inferred from a descriptive categorization of people and their abilities, the result is a misguided moral justification for discrimination and distorted power relations.[11]

7. Conclusion

The original role of bioethics was to engage in debates on ethical issues and values related to biosciences and to life (and death) in general, without indoctrinating or promoting specific ethical positions, unless those positions were themselves critically analyzed and examined. For this, analytical philosophical reflection on the issues of definitions, arguments, and logic was needed. The problems in finding a commonly agreed definition of "bioethics" have, however, gradually led away from reflective philosophical analysis which could have, among other things, helped in finding consistent legal guidelines and policy recommendations.

Instead, today we can detect two main polarized ways of doing "bioethics": abstract theoretical speculation detached from reality on the one hand, and political pragmatism on the other. In order to build a bridge between these extremes, there is a need to bring reflection and argumentation back to bioethics, in a manner that does not turn the discipline into an abstract and over-intellectualized philosophical game that has nothing to do with the context in which ethical questions arise. Bioethics should not go to the other extreme either and take a strong relativist stance that confuses ethical decision-making with unsupported "opinionism" based on a naively pragmatic approach that compares making ethical choices with choosing between flavors of ice-cream. Anthropologists can help us to see the cultural embeddedness of our ethical theory, but we still need philosophical reflection and logic to make sense out of entangled arguments and confusion in the use of concepts, and to understand the differences in our values. If we want to have meaningful bioethical inquiry, we need to focus more on critical philosophical analysis of ethics within the scope of life sciences. This includes the analytical testing of the plausibility of the suggested definitions and of the arguments based on these definitions. Perhaps a good place to start would be with the definition of "bioethics" itself.

NOTES

1. Patrick J. Hurley, *A Concise Introduction to Logic* (Belmont, CA: Wadsworth, Thomson Learning, 2000), pp. 92–93.

2. Ronald Munson and David Conway, *Basics of Reasoning* (Belmont, CA: Wadsworth, Thomson Learning, 2001), pp. 92–93.

3. Hurley, *A Concise Introduction to Logic*, p. 97.

4. Yaman Ors, *Defining Bio-Ethics*, http://www.biopolitics.gr/HTML/PUBS/VOL5/html/ors_tur.htm

5. Ors, *Defining Bio-Ethics*, http://www.biopolitics.gr/HTML/PUBS/VOL5/html/ors_tur.htm

6. Bioethics Council, *Defining Bioethics*, http://www.bioethics.org.nz/about-bioethics/defining.html; Daniel Callahan and Sissela Bok (eds.), *Ethical Teaching in Higher Education* (New York: Plenum Publishing Customer Service, 1980); Dianne N. Irving, "What is 'Bioethics'?" http://www.lifeissues.net/writers/irv/irv_36whatisbioethics01.html; "Nature Genetics Editorial: Defining a New Bioethic," *Nature Genetics* 28 (2001), pp. 297–298, doi:10.1038/91034, http://www.nature.com/ng/journal/v28/n4/full/ng0801_297.html.

7. Matti Häyry and Tuija Takala, "What is Bioethics All About? A Start," *Scratching the Surface of Bioethics*, eds. Matti Häyry and Tuija Takala (Amsterdam and New York: Rodopi, 2003), pp. 1–7; James Dwyer, "Teaching Global Bioethics," *Bioethics*, 17:5–6 (2003), pp. 432–446; Rosemarie Tong, "Feminism and Feminist Bio-ethics: The Search for a Measure of Unity in a Field with Rich Diversity," *New Review of Bioethics*, 1:1 (2003), pp. 85–100.

8. Matti Häyry, *Playing God: Essays on Bioethics* (Helsinki: Helsinki University Press, 2001).

9. Helen Longino, *Science and Social Knowledge* (Princeton: Princeton University Press, 1990); Deborah G. Mayo, *Acceptable Evidence: Science and Values in Risk Management.* (Oxford: Oxford University Press, 1991).

10. Sean Murphy, *Establishment Bioethics*, www.catholiceducation.org/articles/medical_ethics/me0065.html.

11. Michel Foucault, *Madness and Civilization: A History of Insanity in the Age of Reason* (New York: Vintage Books, 1965); Michel Foucault, *The Birth of the Clinic: Archaelogy of Medical Perception* (New York: Random House, 1973).

Two

ETHICS BEYOND APPLICATION

Sven Ove Hansson

1. Introduction

Three common approaches to area-specific ethics are discussed, namely professional, organizational, and applied ethics. It is concluded that they all have serious shortcomings. We need a unified ethical discipline in which fundamental issues of moral theory are treated in close connection with the many changing contexts in which moral argumentation is needed. Subdisciplines such as healthcare ethics and technoethics should be recognized as drivers, not mere recipients, of theoretical developments in ethics. Several social areas are pointed out that are in need of specialized ethical discussion, but have not yet received it.

A rough overview of the ethical literature can be obtained by searching for ethical key terms in major bibliographies. The Philosopher's Index contains most of the literature in general or theoretical ethics. Medline contains most of the literature in ethics related to medicine and healthcare. Most philosophers will be surprised to learn that the latter bibliography contains around 40 percent more publications with one of the words "ethics," "ethical" or "moral" in its title than Philosopher's Index. (A search in August 2005 showed that Medline, as searched via PubMed, contained 29730 publications with one of these three words in its title. The Philosopher's Index contained 21677 such publications. 19885 of these did not contain "bioethics" or "medical" anywhere in the record. Furthermore, Medline reported 116977 publications with one of the three words "ethics," "ethical" or "moral" anywhere in the record. The Philosopher's Index reported 64653 such entries.)

A study of institutional arrangements will confirm this picture. Three decades ago, academic ethics was seldom found outside of departments of philosophy. Today, many universities have centers or departments devoted to the ethics of some specialized practice, such as a center for bioethics or research ethics. There is a growing number of such specializations: bioethics and healthcare ethics, research ethics, ethics of technology, business ethics, agricultural ethics, etc. These area-specific subdisciplines seem to be growing much faster than traditional moral philosophy.

What is the relation between moral philosophy and area-specific ethics? And what *should* the relation be? It is the purpose of the present contribution to try to answer these questions. I will begin by distinguishing between three (admittedly partly overlapping) approaches to area-specific ethics. I will call them professional ethics, organizational ethics, and applied ethics. In the following three sections, each of them will be somewhat schematically characterized in terms of four variables:

1. *Subject area*: How is the subject area of an area-specific ethical subdiscipline delimited?
2. *Practitioners*: What is the typical educational and professional background of those who practice it?
3. *Mode of operation*: What is the typical activity of these practitioners? (Such as developing or interpreting codes of conduct, writing papers for ethics journals, etc.)
4. *Approach to moral theory*: What is the relation to moral theory?

In section 5, a fourth and hopefully more promising approach, the "unified discipline approach" will be proposed for the reader's consideration.

2. Professional Ethics

The oldest tradition in area-specific ethics is professional ethics, the ethics of professions. The medical profession has discussed ethical issues since antiquity. The second part of the Hippocratic oath shows that many of the ethical concerns of physicians have continuity over the ages. However, medical ethics as an academic discipline emerged only in the 1960s. There is also a fairly long tradition of ethical discussions in the engineering profession. Codes of ethics for engineers were written already in the 19th century. However, engineering ethics was not established as an academic subject until the 1970s. Business ethics, agricultural ethics, and computer ethics emerged in the same period.

Research ethics developed from discussions among scientists after World War II, in part in response to revelations about Nazi experiments on human subjects, in part in response to the nuclear bomb. Several ethical codes for scientists were adopted in the years after the war. Activities in this area receded in the 1950s and 1960s, but increased again in the 1970s as part of a new awareness of potential negative consequences of scientific and technological research.

The *subject-area* of these and other forms of professional ethics is constituted by the ethical responsibilities of a particular profession, such as physicians, research scientists, engineers, business managers, etc. This delimitation has obvious advantages. Each of these professions has responsibilities that can be seen as common concerns for members of the respective profession.

However, this delimitation of areas for ethical analysis also has disadvantages. Professional ethics only develops in those social areas that have a strong and responsible profession. Some social areas with important ethical issues do not answer to that description. One of the best examples of this is traffic safety. This is a subject area with many intricate ethical issues that need careful consideration. However, due to the lack of a unified "traffic safety profession," almost no area-specific ethical discussion has taken place in this area. Other examples are welfare provision, insurance, building and architecture, and foreign aid. We need ethical discussions also about social areas that do not have strong professions who develop ethical principles for their own work.

The *practitioners* of professional ethics have mainly been members of the respective profession, typically active members in various professional societies. An obvious advantage of their involvement is that they have expert knowledge in the respective areas. Hence, physicians know the factual background of issues in medical ethics, and engineers in engineering ethics, etc. On the other hand, their lack of background in moral theory often leads to a lack of depth in the ethical analyses. Only rarely are persons without an education in moral philosophy able to make a thorough ethical analysis that goes beyond already established standpoints and arguments.

Furthermore, when the ethical issues in a subject-area are seen predominantly from the viewpoint of a particular profession, other important aspects and perspectives may be neglected. Hence, the focus on health professionals' perspectives in healthcare ethics has often led to neglect of ethical issues in healthcare management and health insurance management. This is unfortunate since it is often managers and administrators who make the most important priority decisions in healthcare. The dominance of the perspective of healthcare professionals may also have led to neglect of issues that are best seen from the perspective of patients. This became clear to me when I served as an ethicist on a committee for the assessment of treatment and prevention of obesity. When I contacted the patients' organization, they brought up a number of important ethical issues, mostly connected with how obese persons are received in healthcare, that were not mentioned spontaneously by physicians.

Similarly, engineering ethics deals with the responsibilities of engineers, but there are many important ethical issues in technology that do not arise primarily in the activities of engineers. In summary, professional ethics is restricted both in its choice of subject areas and in its perspective on the chosen subject areas.

The typical *mode of operation* of professional ethics is rule-setting. Professional organizations have largely approached ethical problems by developing codes of ethics specifying how members of the profession should behave.

They have often also appointed committees of professionals who give advice to members.

Ethical codes can no doubt be an important factor in the professionaliza-tion of a social activity that needs to be conducted in a competent, responsible, and reasonably standardized fashion. They serve to remind members of a pro-fession of ethical requirements that they should take seriously, and facilitate a discussion of these ethical requirements in terms of general principles. It is interesting to note that Roger Boisjoly, one of the engineers who tried to stop the launch of the Challenger, said eleven years later in an interview that he believed it would have made a difference if he had had an ethical code to refer to when approaching his superiors.[1] However, ethical codes can only solve the simple problems. The more difficult cases in professional ethics are almost invariably dilemmatic situations in which the different parts of a code give contradictory advice. Hence, many codes urge engineers to be loyal to their employers and also to protect the safety of the public. It is not difficult to find cases in which these two recommendations cannot both be fully satisfied. In order to deal with such conflicts, ethical argumentation is needed that goes far beyond what is contained in the code.

The relation of professional ethics to *moral theory* is mostly next to non-existent. Rules for behavior are postulated rather than obtained from extended analysis and argumentation. Such an atheoretical approach does not support a critical analysis of norms or the development of new normative standpoints. Ethical codes, of course, tend to codify established social norms, rather than encourage a critical analysis of these norms.[2] This may lead to a lack of fore-sight. When new technologies are introduced in society, we often do not have socially accepted norms for the regulation of their use.[3] What we then need is a thorough analysis of possible consequences and possible moral approaches.

There is one exception to the atheoretical approach in professional ethics: In medical ethics, "intermediate principles" such as autonomy, non-maleficence, beneficence, and justice have an important role. However, these principles are often used as a creed rather than as tools of analysis, and aware-ness of the potential conflicts between the four principles is often surprisingly low.[4]

3. Organizational Ethics

Just like professions, some large organizations, in particular companies but also for instance universities and funding agencies, adopt ethical codes or poli-cies. This has become much more common in the last decade or so, partly due to the movement for corporate social responsibility.

The *subject area* of organizational ethics is determined by the activities and decisions of the organizations in question. The perspective of high-level decision-makers in these organizations is mostly dominant. This is of course an important perspective for many ethical issues, but from the viewpoint of impartial ethical analysis it is not sufficient. A full ethical account for instance of issues related to the energy sector does not consist only of an account of how energy companies should behave under the current political situation. It should also include a discussion of options that are open to other decision-makers, in particular political decision-makers who have the power to change the rules under which these companies are operating.

The *practitioners* of organizational ethics are typically senior decision-makers in the organization in question, and their advisors. Their knowledge about the organization and its environment are of course valuable in the ethical discussion, but just like the typical practitioners of professional ethics, they usually lack the competence needed for a thorough ethical analysis that goes beyond the codification of established standpoints.

In its *mode of operation*, organizational ethics is very similar to professional ethics. It operates by setting rules, typically in the form of codes of conduct, and by enforcing theses codes within the organization. Its relation to *moral theory* is even less developed than that of professional ethics. There seems to be very little contact between organizational ethics and ethics as an academic discipline. The drawback of this is the same as for professional ethics.

4. Applied Ethics

The term "applied ethics" does not seem to have been common before the 1970s. Today, it is the standard term for area-specific moral philosophy.

In practice, the *subject-area* of applied ethics consists almost entirely of the fields that have been opened up by professional ethics. The majority of philosophers who investigate ethical issues in a specific subject-area have their focus on healthcare and related fields. They often prefer the relatively new term "bioethics" to the older term "medical ethics." (The term "bioethics" was coined by Van Rensselaer Potter II, 1911-2001, in 1970.[5])

Other areas of applied ethics include research, technology, agriculture, and business management. It is striking that philosophers who specialize in applied ethics have very seldom opened up new territory for ethical analysis. Instead, they have followed the trails of the practitioners of professional ethics. (Probably, the major exception is environmental ethics, but that area is not always counted as part of applied ethics.) As already mentioned, there are many other subject areas that have equally important ethical problems as those that have become areas of professional and applied ethics.

The *practitioners* of applied ethics are typically persons with an education in moral philosophy. (There is also a surprising number of persons with a religious background but with little background in—secular or theological—ethics who are taken by themselves and many others to be experts in ethics.)

Education in moral philosophy is of course an essential precondition for the ability to perform ethical analysis. However, not all philosophers have realized that it is also necessary to take the time and trouble to develop a thorough understanding of the particular subject area.[6] The principles that apply to personal moral decisions may not apply in all respects to decision-making in specialized institutions such as hospitals or business companies.

Applied ethics also differs from professional and organizational ethics in its *mode of operation*. Like moral philosophy in general, it operates by analyzing problems and developing and discussing alternative standpoints in moral issues. Its output typically consists of articles presenting analyses and arguments, rather than ethical codes intended to guide practitioners in their decisions.

The most interesting difference concerns our fourth variable, the relation to *moral theory*. Applied ethics has in fact been defined as "the application of an ethical theory to some particular moral problem or set of problems."[7] In order to clarify the meaning of "application" in this context it is instructive to compare applied ethics to other applied disciplines, such as applied mathematics. In applied mathematics, a mathematical theory is used to solve some problem outside of pure mathematics. The theory itself is not changed or significantly extended in the process of its application.[8] It would seem that what is going on in the best works for instance in medical ethics is much more then the application—in this sense—of preexisting moral theory.

Applied ethics can be seen as a branch, or collection of branches, of "applied philosophy". However, not all areas of philosophy that deal with specific subject areas are called "applied." Hence, philosophy of law is not called "applied ethics" and neither is philosophy of science called "applied epistemology." The reason for this is fairly obvious. It is generally recognized that the philosophy of law consists of much more than the application of moral theory to legal problems. Similarly, it is recognized that philosophy of science cannot be successfully conducted by transferring and using theories from epistemology. Instead, philosophers of science develop new theory that may be related to epistemology but is not derivable from it.

In my view, the term "applied" is just as misleading for the specialized ethical disciplines as it would have been for legal philosophy or the philosophy of science. Area-specific ethics needs to go beyond preexisting moral theory, just as philosophy of science has to go beyond general epistemology. It is not a workable procedure to develop a moral theory independently of any concrete issue, and then apply it to concrete issues without revising or amending it.[9] It is, for instance, not advisable to approach healthcare ethics armed with a general moral theory and with a strong conviction that it will solve all the problems that come up. In fact, many of the problems that emerge from ethical studies of medical practice have at most weak connections with the choice between ethical theories such as different variants of deontology or utilitarianism.[10]

Bioethics is an innovation-rich discipline that has produced new insights on personhood, consent, and other issues that are pertinent in all branches of ethics. Excellent examples of this can be found in the work of Matti Häyry.[11] It is not obvious today in which direction the most important influence goes between bioethics and basic or general moral philosophy. Ethical studies of other specialized areas also have the potential for developing the same type of strength. Therefore, the use of the term "applied ethics" for these endeavors is unfortunate. It underestimates their innovative potential and gives them an undeservedly low status among philosophical disciplines.

5. A New Approach

My starting-point for a new approach is very simple: Moral philosophy consists primarily in systematic reflections on how we humans should act in our relations to each other. Our actions do not take place in a vacuum but in a natural and social environment. Since this environment is constantly changing, so is the subject-matter of moral philosophy. Developments in human society constantly provide moral philosophy with new subject-matter. New philosophical problems and problem-areas are created, whereas some of the old ones become obsolete. It is easy to give examples of developments in the previous century that had a deep influence on moral philosophy: the emergency of democracy, racism and the holocaust, the threat of a nuclear war, feminism, destruction of the environment, neurobiology, biotechnology, etc.

Our task, as I see it, is not to produce timeless ethics—we might just as well run after the end of the rainbow—but to develop moral theory in relation to our changing society. Therefore, ethical theory cannot proceed in isolation from the surrounding society. It has to develop with society. It follows from this that the ethical studies of various practices such as healthcare, technology, research, etc., have a much more important role than that of being applications of theory. If we want moral philosophy to keep pace with society, ethical studies of such crucial areas of social development must be drivers, not mere recipients, of theoretical development.

From the viewpoint of disciplinary delimitation, this means that the division between fundamental and "applied" ethics should be given up. What we need is a unified approach in which theory development takes place in much closer contact with analyses of actual ethical problems in society. The unified ethical discipline can be summarized in terms of the same four characteristics that we have used for professional, organizational and applied ethics. Its *subject area* should include all problem areas in modern society that require ethical analysis. Its *practitioners* should be persons with a strong background in moral philosophy, who cooperate closely with natural, medical, technological, social, and behavioral scientists and with practitioners in various social areas. Its *mode of operation* should be to analyze problems and to develop and discuss alternative standpoints in moral issues. Its relation to *moral theory* should be that of driving the development of new moral theory.

Ethics is a large research area, and the proposed unified discipline will be so large that specializations are necessary. For want of a better term I propose to use the term "specialized ethics" to denote ethical studies that have their focus on a particular social area. Obviously, health ethics should be one such specialty. This term is preferable to "medical ethics" that has a too strong connection to the profession-oriented perspective on health and disease. As already indicated, ethical issues that lie outside the purview of the medical and nursing professions are worth more attention than what they have usually obtained in ethical studies of healthcare. This includes large-scale economic decisions on healthcare, access to enabling technologies, strategic decisions in the development of new medical technologies, etc.[12]

Another important area for specialized ethics is the ethical study of technology. Instead of the term "engineering ethics," with its strong focus on the perspective of the engineering profession, I propose that the term "technoethics" be used do denote this area of research. Since technology is pivotal in social change, moral philosophy cannot deal adequately with the ethical problems of our changing society without making technoethics a central aspect of the discipline, rather than the marginalized application area that it is today.

6. Conclusion

The four approaches are summarized in *Table 1*. In conclusion, the approaches described here as professional, organizational, and applied ethics all have serious shortcomings. They are all limited in the scope of their subject-areas. Professional ethics is concerned with the ethical problems of certain professions and organizational ethics with those of certain organizations. Applied ethics has seldom broken new ground, but instead limited its interest to the areas previously opened up by professional ethics.

Both professional and organizational ethics typically have an atheoretical approach that limits their capacity for innovativeness. Applied ethics has stronger connections to moral theory. However, the theory-applying approach of applied ethics is too limited and needs to be replaced by a more ambitious, theory-developing approach.

What we need is a unified ethical discipline in which fundamental issues are treated in close connection with the many changing contexts in which moral argumentation is needed—rather than in illusory timelessness and contextlessness.

	Professional ethics	*Organizational ethics*	*Applied ethics*	*The unified discipline*
Subject area	Responsibilities of particular professions	Responsibilities of particular organizations	Responsibilities of particular professions	All problem areas in need of ethical analysis
Practitioners	Members of the respective professions	Decision-makers in the respective organizations	Moral philosophers	Moral philosophers
Mode of operation	Rule-setting	Rule-setting	Analysis and arguments	Analysis and arguments
Approach to theory	Atheoretical	Atheoretical	Theory-applying	Theory-developing

Table 1. A summary of the approaches to area-specific ethics outlined in the text.

NOTES

1. Elizabeth Kane, "Is PE License a Boon to Ethics in Industry?" *Engineering Times*, 19:3 (March 1997), p. 1.
2. Ellen Klein, "The One Necessary Condition for a Successful Business Ethics Course: The Teacher Must Be a Philosopher," *Business Ethics Quarterly*, 8 (1998), pp. 561–574.

3. W. F. Ogburn (ed.), *Social Change With Regard to Cultural and Original Nature* (New York: Dell Publishing Company, 1966); James Moor, "What is Computer Ethics?" *Metaphilosophy*, 16 (1985), pp. 266–275.

4. Tuija Takala, "What Is Wrong with Global Bioethics? On the Limitations of the Four Principles Approach," *Cambridge Quarterly of Healthcare Ethics*, 10 (2001), pp. 72–77.

5. V. R. Potter, "Bioethics: The Science of Survival," *Perspectives in Biology and Medicine*, 14 (1970), pp. 127–153; W. T. Reich, "The Word 'Bioethics': its Birth and the Legacies of Those Who Shaped It," *Kennedy Institute of Ethics Journal*, 4 (1994), pp. 319–35; W. T. Reich, "The Word 'Bioethics': The Struggle Over its Earliest Meanings," *Kennedy Institute of Ethics Journal*, 5 (1995), pp. 19–34.

6. Donald Gotterbarn, "The Moral Responsibility of Software Developers," *Journal of Information Ethics*, 4 (1995), pp. 54–64.

7. Bernard Gert, quoted on pp. 514–515 in Tom Beauchamp, "On Eliminating the Distinction Between Applied Ethics and Ethical Theory," *Monist*, 67 (1984), pp. 514–531.

8. Loretta Kopelman, "What is Applied about 'Applied' Philosophy?" *Journal of Medicine and Philosophy*, 15 (1990), pp. 199–218. See p. 201.

9. Tom Beauchamp, "On Eliminating the Distinction Between Applied Ethics and Ethical Theory"; Alasdair MacIntyre, "Does Applied Ethics Rest on a Mistake?" *Monist*, 67 (1984), pp. 498–513; Sami Pihlström, "Applied Philosophy: Problems and Applications," *International Journal of Applied Philosophy*, 13 (1999), pp. 121–133; Nicholas Rescher, "Is Philosophy a Guide to Life?" *Bowling Green Studies in Applied Philosophy*, 5 (1983), pp. 1–15

10. David Heyd, "Experimenting with Embryos: Can Philosophy Help?" *Bioethics*, 10 (1996), pp. 292–309; Will Kymlicka, "Moral Philosophy and Public Policy: The Case of the New Reproductive Technologies," *Bioethics*, 7 (1993), pp. 1–26; Stephen Toulmin, "The Tyranny of Principles – Regaining the Ethics of Discretion," *Hastings Center Report*, 11 (1981), pp. 31–38.

11. Matti Häyry "Another Look at Dignity," *Cambridge Quarterly of Healthcare Ethics*, 13 (2004), pp. 7–14; Matti Häyry and Tuija Takala, "Genetic Information, Rights, and Autonomy," *Theoretical Medicine and Bioethics*, 22 (2001), pp. 403–414.

12. Sven Ove Hansson, "Implant Ethics," *Journal of Medical Ethics*, 31 (2005), pp. 519–525; Sven Ove Hansson, "The Ethics of Enabling Technology," *Cambridge Quarterly of Healthcare Ethics*, 16 (2007), pp. 257–267.

Three

UTILITARIANISM AND LIBERALISM

Harry Lesser

1. Introduction

In both ethics and politics, perhaps especially in bioethics, one common basic theory, or at least basic approach, is a combination of utilitarianism and liberalism. This way of tackling the problems of bioethics is one that many people, myself included, find attractive: in general, one may expect people who esteem the work of Matti Häyry to find it attractive.[1] But there is a serious question as to whether this approach, however great its emotional appeal, holds together rationally; and whether the two positions, utilitarianism and liberalism, are even compatible with each other. Even some of the people who hold both positions do so by assigning them to different spheres. A good example would be Ronald Dworkin, whose position seems to be that we should tackle political and ethical questions using a utilitarian approach, except where rights are involved, when these "trump" utilitarian considerations.[2] In contrast, there is John Stuart Mill's *On Liberty*, perhaps the classic liberal text, which defends liberalism precisely on utilitarian grounds, and not on grounds of abstract right.[3] This paper seeks to examine, and as a result defend, Mill's view that maximizing personal freedom also in the long term maximizes utility. It also seeks to say something about the consequences of this for bioethics.

2. Defining Utilitarianism and Liberalism

We need to begin with definitions. In general terms utilitarianism is easy to define, as the theory that what is morally right at any given time is that which maximizes happiness or at any rate minimizes suffering. But then the problems start. Do we apply this to actions, to rules for action or to general policies? For the purposes of bioethics we can say that we are essentially concerned with ways of behaving, with systems and policies rather than individual actions. Secondly, do we define happiness in terms of pleasure and pain, or in terms of satisfaction of preferences? Here, I will assume that the theory of utilitarianism has improved as it has developed, and that contemporary utilitarians are right to see satisfaction of preferences as the better option, given that pleasure is not the only thing we want, and pain, however widely defined, not the only thing we seek to avoid. I will also assume that John Harris, for example in his *The Value of Life* (1985), and others are right to conclude both that the preferences of each person are of equal importance and that certain preferences, notably the desires for life and for liberty, must be privileged and regarded as of supreme importance, since if anyone is denied life or liberty they are obviously denied the chance of satisfying any other preferences.[4] The more controversial question, of whether there are other wants or preferences that should be privileged, because they meet the deepest human needs, will be left undecided.

Liberalism can obviously mean very different things. In this paper it will be defined as the theory that all adult members of society should be free to participate in decision making, to compete on equal terms, and to take their own decisions in what concerns themselves entirely or primarily: the first and third of these are particularly relevant to bioethics. (It should be noted that here and elsewhere the words "Liberal" and "Liberalism" have the British, not the American, connotation). Given these definitions, the problem to be addressed is the following: Is the liberal model of health care, in which patients and clients are encouraged to make their own decisions as to what treatment they are given, at all consistent with the utilitarian requirement, that the aim of health care must be to maximize healthy functioning, physical and mental, and minimize disease and pain?

3. Wants, Needs, and Liberalism

Why should liberalism and utilitarianism, thus defined, not be consistent? This is because of two reasons. First, liberalism, as defined above, seems to entail that at least some—not all but some—crucial decisions should be taken according to the choices of individuals, regardless of other considerations. Liberalism, in bioethics as elsewhere, is committed to the existence of individual rights, and to holding that these rights hold irrespective of the consequences. Utilitarianism, in contrast, is committed to the view that there are no absolute rights, and that the general welfare should overrule individual wishes and choices. So it seems that for a liberal, health care should be distributed according to what people want: patients are entitled to the health care that they choose, if it is available. If there is not enough to go round, so to speak (and there never is), it should be a matter of "first come, first served" or, for those liberals who believe in the "free market," of health care going to those able to pay. In contrast, a utilitarian must logically hold that health care must be distributed according to need, or according to an expert assessment of what will do the most good; and this will clearly produce a different distribution from the "liberal" one.

But is liberalism really committed to this? It is committed to holding that medical treatment may not be forced on a person against their will, even if the experts believe it would be beneficial. (The exceptions to this will be discussed later on.) But it is not in any way committed to holding that people are entitled to the treatment that they want, regardless of the claims of others whose condition is more serious, or of the assessment by doctors that the treatment will do no good. Nor is it committed to the view that medical care and resources should be distributed according to the ability to pay. There are liberals who hold both these positions, but they are not essential to liberalism. Notably, they are not part of the liberalism of *On Liberty*. For what Mill holds is that a person should not be compelled to do, or refrain from doing, anything "for their own good," that is, because in the opinion of others it would be to their benefit, or wise, or right; but once their actions harm others there is a duty to intervene.[5] Moreover, all that is involved here is the idea that one should not interfere with what people do when it does no harm to others, or (though Mill himself explicitly rejects this formulation and its implications) the idea that people have a right not to be interfered with in this sphere. There is nothing to suggest that people have any positive right to be provided with what they want simply because they want it. Least of all is this the case when they do harm, even unintentional harm, by taking it, as would be the case if they had a "right" to useless medical treatments, and could take care and resources away from those who would be helped by them. It is also not the case when other people have a greater claim in justice to the resources, for example by being obviously in greater need.

One may add that the ideas that medical resources should be distributed according to the wants of the first-comers, or according to the results of the free market, though they are part of one version of liberalism, are not in fact consistent with its basic principle, that freedom should be maximized. The maximization of freedom requires that the more serious obstacles to it be tackled in preference to the less serious, if one cannot tackle both; in the area of health this means that the more seriously ill take precedence over the less seriously ill, even if this means that the wishes of the less seriously ill are temporarily thwarted. It also requires that inequalities of power be limited; and this in its turn may require that there be limitations both on economic inequality and on how the better off may use their money. There may well be an important place for the free market; but there is no guarantee that every operation of the free market increases overall freedom, or that every limitation on it will diminish freedom. In particular, there are good reasons for thinking that freedom is best served by distributing health care according to need rather than according to the market.[6]

4. Utilitarianism and Individual Rights

So we may say that one supposed reason why utilitarianism and liberalism are incompatible should be rejected. Liberalism does not require us to put the mere desires of one person above the real needs (those things which are actually essential to life or health) of others; and those who think it does may well be subscribing to an ultimately inconsistent liberal theory. But there is a further problem. Liberalism seems to be committed to individual rights, whether by holding that there are moral as well as legal rights or by holding that there are some things, such as life and liberty, which ought to be legally protected everywhere: even Mill, though he rejects any appeal to liberty as an abstract right, elsewhere endorses the general notion of rights.[7] Now this does seem to be incompatible with utilitarianism, for this commits the liberal to holding that some things may not be done to a person whatever the consequences; and the utilitarian is committed to holding that nothing can be excluded totally, if the circumstances warrant it. Thus the utilitarian, it might be said, even if they privilege life, will still have to hold that one life should be taken in order to preserve many lives; whereas the liberal will hold that life may be taken only when the right to life has been forfeited, for example by making a murderous attack.

But it is not clear that the utilitarian has to take this position. There are utilitarians, notably R. M. Hare in his *Moral Thinking* (1981), who have argued, in effect, that though to take one innocent life to save many would be of short-term benefit, long-term human welfare requires us to make such things as life and liberty absolute rights.[8] This is very plausible: given the temptation to those in power to withhold respect even from life and liberty, and the enormous risk of abuse, once one accepts that taking life can be a right in principle, there are excellent grounds for saying that a utilitarian should take exactly the same position as a liberal on this issue, and hold that there should be an absolute right to life, which perhaps can be forfeited but cannot be overridden.

Two objections might be made here. One is that if one takes this view one has refined utilitarianism so much that it has become a different theory. But the claim is that rights to life and liberty (and maybe others) should be maintained because they are necessary for the long-term welfare of humanity; and this is a utilitarian claim. The other objection is the reverse of this, that to base these rights on utilitarian considerations, rather than the mere fact of a person's humanity, is already to abandon liberalism. In one sense of "liberalism" this is true; but then liberalism defined in this way is by definition not compatible with utilitarianism! What we are concerned with is simply the policy of liberalism, particularly in bioethics, and whether this must necessarily be different from a utilitarian policy.

5. The Problem of Paternalism

So far, I have argued that there should be no difference between the way the right to life is viewed by a liberal and by a utilitarian. But what about the right to freedom? This brings us to the second major problem with regard to the compatibility of liberalism and utilitarianism in bioethics, namely the issue of paternalism, as it is commonly called. For it might well be argued that in matters of health care the way to maximize utility is to put decision-making into the hands of the professionals, the doctors, nurses and others, whereas liberalism requires that it be in the hands of the client or patient. We could agree with Mill that a person is by and large a better judge of their own interests than are other people, however well-intentioned; but this seems to be true only when expertise is not involved, as it is here. One might add to this, though controversially, that many people who require medical treatment are, of course, ill, and even physical illness, let alone mental illness, warps the judgment: "A sick man is but a child" (Watson to Holmes in "The dying detective"). The crucial argument, though, is that in order to maximize utility decisions need to be made by those with knowledge, rather than by the laity.

The first reply one can make to this is that the decisions about medical treatment which a person has to take often need to be based on non-medical as well as medical considerations: the best thing to do is not always what is medically best. For example, one might postpone treatment, even if the delay increased the risk of failure, in order to complete something one has a duty to do, or even simply very much wants to do. One might refuse the best treatment (the one most likely to succeed) because it involved physical disfigurement. One might prefer to live with pain than to endure the loss of mental alertness caused by pain-killers. These examples, and many others, indicate that the medical situation is only part of what has to be taken into account when deciding what to do, even when deciding what to do with regard to medical treatment. This cannot be done if, as on the old model of medical care, the doctor takes all the decisions on the patient's behalf. It can be done, and there is then a better chance of utility being maximized, if the "new" model is used, where the professional presents the options to the client, who then makes a (hopefully) informed choice or else explicitly decides to leave the decision to the doctor. (Of course, neither method is foolproof.)

The situation is actually more complicated. Not only may the medically best option not be the overall best option, given the patient's tastes and wants, and their perception of what is their duty; there may be no medically best option. Medicine has at least three aims—to maintain, or restore, the functioning of the body and its organs, to relieve pain and suffering, and to prolong life. These very often go together: curing a serious disease with antibiotics, for example, will achieve them all. But sometimes they do not, as in the example above, where the relief of pain involved some loss of mental alertness. In the previous paragraph I treated this as an example of the medical versus the non-medical, but it could be treated as an example of a situation in which one cannot even have everything that is medically valuable, and must make a choice. And the choice has to be a personal one: no one is in a position to tell the patient that one decision is better than the other. One might respect the person who chooses mental alertness at the expense of pain, but one cannot say the other person is wrong. The same can be said about those terrible situations in which the choice is between death, on the one hand, and life with unrelievable suffering, on the other. There are arguments for and against euthanasia, but there is certainly no ground for saying that the doctors are the best judges of whether a person's life is or is not worth living. They are the best judges of some of the relevant considerations, such as whether a cure is likely, or whether the pain can be relieved, but that is not the same thing.

So we may say, first, that the best course of action is not necessarily what is medically best, and secondly, that there is not always a "medically best" course of action. The situation is further complicated by the fact that what have to be weighed up are possible or probable risks and benefits, rather than features of the actual situation. Thus, one available treatment for a particular condition might offer total cure if things went right, at the risk of permanent harm if they did not. Another treatment might offer only a partial cure, but with a very high chance of success and little or no risk of harm in the event of failure. One can here multiply examples, since there are at least four variables; possible degree of success; likelihood of success; seriousness of the consequences of failure; and the likelihood of failure. But the common factor is that very often there are no right answers, it is a matter of what risks a person chooses to run for what benefits. The expert can say what is likely to happen in each case and what the risks are, but they cannot say what is actually the best thing to do, since there is no best thing to do—only a choice to be made.

So even on utilitarian grounds the choice should still be left to the client/patient, to the person who knows where the shoe pinches, as Mill might have put it. There are exceptions to this: children; those who are unconscious, drugged, drunk or delirious, and the seriously mentally ill or mentally impaired. (Age is not in itself a factor, though the incidence of some mental illnesses, such as Alzheimer's Disease, does increase with age). But all these cases are exceptions for liberalism just as much as for utilitarianism: no liberal would maintain that a person who is incompetent to make decisions should nevertheless have the right to make them. There are sometimes great problems in deciding when and in what areas a person is not competent, but these problems exist whatever one's basic position. And it is true, as a matter of fact, that because of the importance liberals attach to freedom, they are particularly reluctant to declare people incompetent. Thomas Szasz, for example, specifically connects his denial that there is such a thing as mental illness with his libertarian political views.[9] Nevertheless, if the argument of this paper, and of Mill, is correct, a consistent utilitarian should adopt the liberal position, of assuming competence in adults unless there is a definite reason to believe it is lacking, and allowing the competent to make their own decisions in what concerns them solely, or primarily and most immediately.

6. Classical and Modern Liberalism

But although the above argument is the main utilitarian argument for liberalism in bioethics, there is another, very different but still important, one to be found in Mill. This is the argument that having to think for oneself and make one's own decisions develops both the intellect and the character, makes people both sharp-witted and self-reliant. In their turn these qualities benefit both the individuals themselves and society in general. Mill points out at some length how hard it is for a society to accomplish anything without citizens who have such qualities. Now this is not a subsidiary point: it has implications both for the version of liberalism we should adopt and for its application to bioethics.

The thing to be aware of at this point is the considerable difference between Mill's liberalism and what is often currently taken to be liberalism, although it is only one version of it. According to this version of modern liberalism, the function of the State is to protect its citizens from external and internal threats and to provide a "safety net" for those unable to look after themselves: it has no business to require, or even to encourage, its citizens to adopt any particular view of the good life, or even to require them to help each other, beyond making their contributions, whether via taxation or military service, to such things as common defense. As a corollary, the only duties of citizens are to do their fellow-citizens no harm and to make their contribution. They may choose to combine with other public-spirited people to do things of public benefit, and they may be praised for so doing; but provided they do not interfere with their fellow-citizens they fail in no duty if they simply pursue their private goals or interests.

Now this is not Mill's liberalism. For Mill the State is as much entitled to require its citizens to do positive good as it is to prevent them from doing harm. It is true that in practice, as Mill says in the last chapter of *On Liberty*, this should be the exception rather than the rule.[10] There are good reasons for this—the difficulty of enforcing it in practice, the resentment the attempt to enforce it may cause, the interference with privacy it might require, and the uncertainty as to what really is good and beneficial (it is much easier to be sure that something is harmful). But in principle, for Millian liberalism, it is wrong to force people to do things for their own good, but not wrong in principle to force them to benefit other people. Nevertheless, one main reason for not in practice forcing them to do this would be the utilitarian one that these things may be done a lot better if they are done voluntarily.

Also, even when force should not be used, encouragement and persuasion may and should. Even for a person's own good, though one may not use force, one should use persuasion and remonstration.[11] Equally, or even more, one should educate people to be public-spirited: this is not only what one should be doing as a citizen, but also to one's advantage as a person: Mill says, rightly, in the first chapter of *Utilitarianism*, that a prime cause of people's unhappiness is "caring for no one but themselves."[12] The Millian ideal is not an "atomized" society, in which people pursue their own ends, singly or in groups, being concerned with others only as regards doing them no harm. It is an ideal of everyone sharing in the advancement of the public good. The "negative freedom" that Mill advocates has the aim not simply of letting people decide for themselves the things they are best placed to decide, but also of seeing to it that those who take part in public affairs—which, in an ideal state would be everybody—are intelligent, alert and self-reliant, and thus fit to take part in public activities and public decision-making. And it is reasonable to think that this, if even partially obtainable, would be a better and happier society than the "atomized" one.

This has an interesting, though not immediately obvious, consequence for current bioethics. It is widely agreed that the old paternalistic model, of the doctor or other professional taking the decisions on behalf of the patient/client, should be where possible abandoned. But what should take its place? It is often supposed that the alternative model should be that of the patient as consumer, who is to be told the likely consequences of various options and then allowed to make a (hopefully) informed choice. But if the preceding argument is correct, this model connects with an essentially impoverished version of liberalism, involving a society essentially concerned with private interests and goals. The model that connects with the richer version of liberalism that was, as we have seen, advocated by Mill, and, as we have also seen, is justified on utilitarian grounds, is the "partnership" model. In this the patient is required to be not a passive consumer of services but a person actively taking responsibility for their own health, and working with the professionals to achieve, maintain or restore it, according to what is needed and what is possible. The full implications of this need to be worked out; but one may suggest that this is the way forward.

To summarize and repeat: Utilitarianism, if this means maximizing long-term human welfare, is, if the arguments of this paper, and of its inspirer, Mill, are correct, not only compatible with liberalism but can be achieved only through liberal policies. But the kind of liberalism of which this is true is the "rich" liberalism of Mill, and not the "debased" version of some contemporary thinkers. This has the consequence that in bioethics the paternalistic model should indeed be seen as to be replaced. But it should be replaced not by the consumer model but by the partnership one.

NOTES

1. Matti Häyry, *Liberal Utilitarianism and Applied Ethics* (London and New York: Routledge, 1994).

2. Ronald Dworkin, *A Matter of Principle* (Oxford: Oxford University Press, 1985).

3. John Stuart Mill, *On Liberty* in *On Liberty and other Writings* (Cambridge: Cambridge University Press, 1989), esp. early chapter 1.

4. John Harris, *The Value of Life* (London: Routledge, 1985).

5. Mill, *On Liberty*, chapter 1.

6. E. F. Carritt, "Liberty and Equality," *Political Philosophy*, ed. Anthony Quinton (Oxford: Oxford University Press, 1967).

7. John Stuart Mill, *Utilitarianism*, ed. George Sher (Hackett Publishing Company, 2nd ed., 2002), chapter 5.

8. Richard Mervyn Hare, *Moral Thinking: Its Levels, Methods and Point* (Oxford: Oxford University Press, 1981).

9. Thomas Stephen Szasz, *Ideology and Insanity: Essays on the Psychiatric Dehumanization of Man* (Penguin Books, 1974).

10. Mill, *On Liberty*, chapter 5.

11. *Ibid.*, chapter 1.

12. Mill, *Utilitarianism*, chapter 5.

Part Two

HOW TO DO BIOETHICS?

Four

THE UNBEARABLE LIGHTNESS OF BIOETHICAL PRINCIPLES

Veikko Launis

If there is such a thing as the truth about the subject matter of ethics—the truth, we might say, about the ethical—why is there any expectation that it should be simple? In particular, why should it be conceptually simple, using only one or two ethical concepts, such as *duty* or *good state of affairs*, rather than many? Perhaps we need as many concepts to describe it as we find we need, and no fewer.[1]

1. Introduction: Metaphysical and Normative Lightness

In the past two decades or so, a mode of theorizing commonly known as "principlism" or a "principle-based approach" has been the dominant approach in bioethics. As Donald C. Ainslie points out, the label "principlism" was originally meant to be derogatory, but became embraced by its defenders.[2] In the form it has come to be known, principlism is usually characterized by adopting a limited number of *prima facie* binding bioethical principles which are then individually specified and balanced against each other when a specific moral problem is discussed. The derivation of the principles, the number of principles, and the specification and balancing methods differ depending on the interpretation.[3]

Though there are different principlist theories, principlism is most commonly characterized by citing four so-called "midlevel" principles—*respect for autonomy* (the obligation to respect and promote the decision-making capacities of autonomous individuals), *nonmaleficence* (the obligation to avoid the causation of harm), *beneficence* (the obligation to provide benefits and balance benefits against risks), and *justice* (obligations of fairness and non-discrimination in the distribution of benefits and risks). The principles are called "midlevel principles," since they are located below moral theories and above moral rules, the general idea being that principles follow from moral theories and, in turn, generate more specific rules that are then used to make moral judgments concerning particular cases.[4] The idea is that these principles can (one way or another) provide the proper justificatory framework for bio-ethics and be used as a method for resolving bioethical issues.

It is not surprising that principlism has so often been attacked by academic philosophers and professional (clinical) bioethicists, because the term "midlevel" already in itself suggests a compromise between two key spheres of ethics—theory and practice. However, as Allen Buchanan, Dan Brock, Norman Daniels and Daniel Wikler have remarked, to a large extent the critics of principlism have been attacking a view "that is at worst a strawman and at best a vulgarization of the framework for analysis advanced most prominently by James Childress and Tom L. Beauchamp in various editions of their influential book *Principles of Biomedical Ethics*."[5] In this chapter, I will attempt to show that, if taken seriously, principlism can provide a defensible normative framework in bioethics. Because there is at present considerable controversy about the proper theory and methodology for bioethics, it would be unrealistic to hope to resolve these complex issues here.[6] My modest aim is to raise certain philosophical questions about the (metaphysical and normative) adequacy and sufficiency of the principle-based approach.

2. The Varieties of Bioethical Problems

The extent to which a bioethical issue can usefully be discussed by reference to midlevel principles depends, of course, on the kind of issue it is. For the purposes of the present discussion, four kinds of issues may be distinguished.[7]

Firstly, some issues are, or turn out to be, controversial largely because relevant empirical facts are in dispute. These may be called *empirical ethical problems*. A possible example of this category of issues is the question whether the development and cultivation of genetically modified crops should be permitted because of the risk they pose to the environment and people's health. It should be no surprise that the contribution of moral philosophers to discussions of these issues is often very limited.

Secondly, there are issues that may be characterized as *conflicts between principles*. A classic example would be the question as to whether a woman's right to autonomy and self-protection overrides her unborn child's (assumed) right to life in the case of abortion. Issues of this kind are *genuine* ethical problems in the sense that the moral conflict may remain even when the empirical facts are clear and accepted by all parties involved in the disagreement.

Thirdly, there are issues that are most properly called *relevance* or *interpretation problems*. These are characteristically raised by novel technologies and new scientific inventions. We may speak of a relevance problem when we are confronted with a new situation in which our traditional principles do not seem to apply very well and we are unable to see what features of the situation are relevant to its moral appraisal. To give an example, whether experiments in human reproductive cloning techniques should be permitted is largely a relevance problem, because we do not know what is morally speaking involved in the development of such techniques.

Finally, there are issues that may be characterized as *demand-for-reason problems*. There is a demand-for-reason problem when we consider a certain practice to be morally acceptable (for instance, using genetically modified mice as cancer models) or unacceptable (for instance, waiving the informed consent rule in the context biobanks) but are unable to specify on what morally relevant grounds it may be considered so, even though there is a morally justifiable demand for providing such a ground.

These four categories are, of course, interconnected and may occur either simultaneously or in succession. To take an example, experiments in human reproductive cloning techniques may be seen to constitute a demand-for-reason problem as well, because such experiments are prohibited by common consent without there being any well-articulated moral ground for such a prohibition.[8] As soon as such grounds can be articulated, objections to them will be raised and human cloning techniques are likely to constitute new empirical ethical problems as well as new conflicts between principles.

3. The Method

How, then, can such problems be resolved? The above discussion suggests that *there is no one thing we can do that is always central to solving an ethical problem for there is no one paradigmatic ethical problem*.[9] Nevertheless, something more constructive and more general needs to be said. The central methodological assumption here is that the coherentist view of moral justification offers the best guidance for bioethical issues. (There are also other methods of moral justification within the principle-based approach.[10]) By coherentism I mean the process of working back and forth between our considered moral judgments about particular situations and general moral rights and principles that cover these situations and help to explain our intuitive beliefs about them. (Considered moral judgments are judgments which we affirm with great confidence and without hesitation. Some such judgments are very specific, whereas others are more general. No matter how general, considered judgments are not to be seen as self-evident nor necessary truths, but as open to revision—and sometimes even rejection—in the process of reflection. Considered moral judgments have some modest degree of epistemic priority simply because some sources of error and distortion, such as the agent's being upset or frightened, have been eliminated from the deliberation process.) The key idea underlying this method is that "we test various parts of our system of moral beliefs against other parts of our general system of beliefs, seeking coherence among the widest set of moral and nonmoral beliefs by revising and refining them at all levels."[11] For example, we might test the appropriateness of the informed consent doctrine in the context of human biobanks by asking whether we can accept its implications in this particular context and whether it accounts for the particular cases discussed within this context better than alternative principles.

Our considered moral judgments and beliefs about particular cases count in this process. Such judgments have justificatory weight for at least two reasons. Firstly, they can be referred to when applying more specific bioethical methods, such as reasoning by analogy and slippery slope arguments.[12] Secondly, they provide what Norman Daniels has called "provisional fixed points," which makes them usable not only in the process of "testing" and reformulating midlevel principles but also in attempts to resolve conflicts between such principles.

I take general philosophical reasoning (including metaphysics, philosophy of mind, rational decision-making, etc.) to be an elementary part of this method. Such reasoning is needed for example when we address the largely discussed question as to whether there is something morally special about genetic medical information as compared with non-genetic medical information. One answer to this question is the (partly) metaphysical claim that genetic information is morally exceptional because genetic (disease) characteristics are more important to our "essential core identity" than non-genetic (disease) characteristics.[13]

The principle-based approach, according to the method sketched above, is not simply a list of midlevel principles, as the principlist caricature would have it. On the contrary, the pluralistic principlist theory has a more complex basic structure than most traditional monistic theories, which regard all midlevel principles as reducible to one basic moral principle. The principlist theory is also much more complex in application than most traditional theories. These complexities, I believe, are not a weakness but rather a virtue of the theory, since complex issues require complex theories and sophisticated methods for their resolution.

4. A Modest Defense of the Framework

Of course, the above sketched framework is not without its problems, and it has many viable competitors.[14] In the remainder of this chapter I clarify my methodology and dismiss a number of possible objections.

By far the best-argued attacks on principlism have come from two sources: K. Danner Clouser and Bernard Gert (the "deductivist" side), and Earl R. Winkler (the "casuistic" side). Let me examine these arguments in turn.

A. "The Mantra of Principles" Objection

According to the Clouser and Gert criticism, the principle-based approach is both misleading and inadequate because

> [i]t lacks systematic unity, and thus creates both practical and theoretical problems. Since there is no moral theory that ties the "principles" together, there is no unified guide to action which generates clear, coherent, comprehensive, and specific rules for action nor any justification of those rules. ... In principlism each discussion of a "principle" is really an eclectic discussion that emphasizes a different type of ethical theory, so that a single unified theory is not only not presented, but the need for such a theory is completely obscured. Rather we are given a number of insights, considerations, and theories, along with instructions to use whichever one or combination of them seems appropriate to the user. But what is needed is that which tells us what actually is appropriate in a consistent and universal fashion. Certainly the "principles" themselves, as portrayed by principlism do not do so. Rather, it is a moral theory that is needed to unify all the "considerations" raised by the "principles" and thus to help us determine what is appropriate.[15]

The objection is, in other words, that the midlevel principles lack any systematic relationship to each other, and they often conflict with each other. These conflicts are unresolvable, since there is no unified moral theory from which they are all derived. There is no priority ranking, nor is there any specified procedure to be used in resolving particular cases of conflicts between the principles. Principlism often has two or even three competing principles involved in a given case. In Clouser and Gert's view, this is tantamount to using two or three conflicting moral theories to resolve a problem.

As a response, one should recognize that Clouser and Gert's objection presupposes two things. Firstly, it presupposes the optimistic metaethical belief that resolving ethical issues in a "consistent and universal fashion" is almost always possible. Secondly, it presupposes the (related) metaethical assumption that in genuine moral conflicts "theory always comes first." To my mind, both beliefs are suspect.

To take the former presupposition first, when moral principles (and theories) are in conflict, making progress is not possible unless one has at hand some specific procedure for establishing priorities among them. I have already argued that such a method exists. It is essential to see, however, that while the method (coherentist philosophical argumentation) frequently yields to a priority among the conflicting moral principles and ideas, there are—and will continue to be—cases where the conflicts are more or less unresolvable.

This, however, should not be interpreted as meaning that the principlist theory is impractical or incomplete. Such a conclusion would be warranted only if it were the case that in moral conflicts "theory always comes first." As far as I can see, this is far from being the case. A little reflection will show us why.

Consider first the two different meanings which, according to Raymond Devettere, the word "principle" has had in ethics.

> First, the word "principle" has sometimes designated what is the begin-ning or the source of the ethical theory itself. *Principles so understood are founding or originative principles*, and they are not derived from, nor defended by, moral theories. Rather, moral theories are derived from, and defended by founding principles. Second, the word "principle" has also designated a norm for a standard used to make particular moral judg-ments about right and wrong. *Principles are thus normative or "action-guides,"* and they are derived from, or at least defended by, moral theo-ries.[16]

In my opinion, both uses are correct and may occur simultaneously. That is to say, moral principles play a dual role in bioethics (and ethics). On the one hand, they serve as general normative guides or prescriptions which are speci-fied and (at least to some extent) defended by moral theories. In this sense, principles are properly described as "midlevel." On the other hand, principles constitute the source or the beginning of moral theory, since they are expres-sions of what John Stuart Mill called in his *Utilitarianism* "ultimate moral ends." As Mill himself was prepared to admit, "questions of ultimate ends do not admit of proof" (in the ordinary use of the term).[17] In this sense, principles are properly described as "toplevel."

As soon as we adopt this approach to moral theories, we recognize that in genuinely problematic cases—particularly in cases of conflicts between ulti-mate principles—moral theories may not be able to resolve the questions with-out there being a loss of value on the way. The reason for this is simple: moral theories cannot necessarily get behind (or above) ultimate moral principles and values.

So, then, it seems that sometimes when genuine conflicts between ulti-mate moral principles occur, there is a considerable lack of unity *in morality (and life) itself*, a lack of unity which no moral theory can eliminate without distorting the actual moral landscape.

B. "The Case-Insensitivity" Objection

The second attack on principlism comes from Earl R. Winkler. He writes:

> Even including the sophistication of reflective equilibrium theory, [the principle-based approach] remains open to the charge of being seriously mistaken. It can be said to leave out of account the very complex processes of *interpretation* that constitute our moral understanding both of cases and of principles. Most importantly, within the complex realities of practice, it is dominantly the interpretation of cases that informs our understanding of principles rather than principles guiding the resolution of difficult cases. All or most of the real work in actual moral reasoning and decision-making is case-driven rather than theory-driven. Therefore, [the principlist theory], even when amended by the methodology of reflective equilibrium, sustains the illusion that bioethics is essentially or primarily a matter of constructing and applying principles when in fact it is almost anything but this.[18]

Winkler is surely right that bioethical principles do not interpret themselves and that "case-sensitive" moral reasoning is needed. In addition to particular cases (often occurring in the clinical context), there are also difficulties in interpreting *kinds* of cases, especially regarding novel issues that are generated by rapidly changing human gene and biotechnology. Above, I have described such difficulties as *relevance problems* (or interpretation problems). Genuine relevance problems, I believe, are likely to cause difficulties to *any* theory of bioethics, no matter what its structure and content. In this regard, there is nothing special about principlism.

When it comes to interpretation itself, it seems to me that the methodology sketched above provides the kind of specificity needed. It goes much deeper than Winkler gives us to understand. First of all, considered moral judgments may undeniably force case-sensitive (and context-specific) modifications and adjustments in our commitment to bioethical principles sometimes. (This may happen, for example, when the traditional doctrine of individual informed consent is explored in the context of human gene and biobanks.) Secondly, as James Childress has pointed out, the principlist theory "can recognize the importance of settled cases, so-called paradigm cases about which there is a wide moral consensus, and can reason analogically from such cases to new or controversial ones."[19] Quite often, the resolution of such novel or controversial cases deepens and broadens our understanding of the relevant bioethical principles and their applicability.

5. Conclusion

To conclude, then, it seems to me that the above criticism fails to show why the principle-based approach should be regarded as theoretically inadequate. By drawing attention to the pluralistic metaethical background of the principle-based approach, I have proposed an interpretation of this approach which seems to be immune to the most serious attacks on it. In the light of my analysis, the particular kind of lightness of bioethical principles, resulting from the fact that there is a plurality of values and principles which can conflict with one another, and which are not reducible to one another, seems quite bearable. Needless to say, as any bioethical theory, the principlist theory can show its ultimate theoretical and practical adequacy only when it concerns itself with real bioethical disputes.

ACKNOWLEDGEMENTS

I am grateful to Olli Koistinen and Juha Räikkä for helpful comments, criticism, and suggestions.

NOTES

1. Bernard Williams, *Ethics and the Limits of Philosophy* (Cambridge: Harvard University Press, 1985), p. 17.
2. Donald C. Ainslie, "Principlism," *Encyclopedia of Bioethics*, 3rd edition, Vol. 4, ed. Stephen G. Post (New York: Macmillan Reference, 2004), p. 2098.
3. Søren Holm, "Principles of Health Care Ethics: Solution or Problem?" *Genes and Morality: New Essays*, eds. Veikko Launis, Juhani Pietarinen and Juha Räikkä (Amsterdam and Atlanta: Rodopi, 1999), p. 51; James F. Childress, "A Principle-Based Approach," *A Companion to Bioethics*, eds. Helga Kuhse and Peter Singer (Oxford: Blackwell, 1998), pp. 61–63; Michael Quante and Andreas Vieth, "Defending Principlism Well Understood," *Journal of Medicine and Philosophy*, 27 (2002), pp. 621–649.
4. See Tom L. Beauchamp and James F. Childress, *Principles of Biomedical Ethics* (New York and Oxford: Oxford University Press, 4th ed., 1994), ch. 1; Childress, "A Principle-Based Approach," pp. 61–71.
5. Allen Buchanan, Dan W. Brock, Norman Daniels and Daniel Wikler, *From Chance to Choice: Genetics and Justice* (New York: Cambridge University Press, 2000), p. 375.
6. *Cf.* Matti Häyry, *Liberal Utilitarianism and Applied Ethics* (London: Routledge, 1994), ch. 4.
7. See Juha Räikkä and Veikko Launis, "Geenietiikka," *Sosiaalilääketieteellinen Aikakauslehti*, 28 (1991): 197–206; see also Bernard Williams, *Moral Luck: Philosophical Papers 1973–1980* (Cambridge: Cambridge University Press, 1981), ch. 5; James D. Wallace, *Moral Relevance and Moral Conflict* (Ithaca: Cornell University

Press, 1988), ch. 1; Peter Singer, *Practical Ethics*, 2nd edition (Cambridge: Cambridge University Press, 1993).

8. *E.g.*, Matti Häyry, "Philosophical Arguments For and Against Human Reproductive Cloning," *Bioethics*, 17 (2003), pp. 447–459.

9. *Cf.* Wibren van der Burg, "Reflective Equilibrium as a Dynamic Process," *Applied Ethics and Reflective Equilibrium*, ed. Bo Petersson (Linköping: Linköpings Universitet, Centre for Applied Ethics, 2000), pp. 78–79.

10. *E.g.*, Heike Schmidt-Felzmann, "Pragmatic Principles—Methodological Pragmatism in the Principle-Based Approach to Bioethics," *Journal of Medicine and Philosophy*, 28 (2003), pp. 581–596.

11. See Buchanan et al., *From Chance to Choice*, p. 376; see also Norman Daniels, *Justice and Justification: Reflective Equilibrium in Theory and Practice* (Cambridge: Cambridge University Press, 1996), chs 1–8.

12. See Alan H. Goldman, *Moral Knowledge* (London: Routledge, 1988), p. 160; Veikko Launis, "Human Gene Therapy and the Slippery Slope Argument," *Medicine, Health Care and Philosophy*, 5 (2002), pp. 169–179.

13. *E.g.*, my "Genetic and Nongenetic Medical Information: Is There a Moral Difference in the Context of Insurance?" *Reconfiguring Nature: Issues and Debates in the New Genetics*, ed. Peter Glasner (Aldershot: Ashgate, 2004), pp.185–202.

14. *E.g.*, Matti Häyry's "liberal utilitarianism" in his *Liberal Utilitarianism and Applied Ethics*, esp. chs 3–4; see also his "What the Fox Would Have Said, Had He Been a Hedgehog: On the Methodology and Normative Approach of John Harris's Wonderwoman and Superman," *Genes and Morality: New Essays*, pp. 11–19.

15. K. Danner Clouser and Bernard Gert, "A Critique of Principlism," *The Journal of Medicine and Philosophy*, 15 (1990): 219–236. See also Ronald M. Green, "Method in Bioethics: A Troubled Assessment," *The Journal of Medicine and Philosophy*, 15 (1990): 179–197; Ronald M. Green, Bernard Gert and K. Danner Clouser, "The Method of Public Morality versus the Method of Principlism," *The Journal of Medicine and Philosophy*, 18 (1993): 477–489; K. Danner Clouser and Bernard Gert, "Morality vs. Principlism," *Principles of Health Care Ethics*, ed. Raanan Gillon (Chichester: John Wiley & Sons, 1994), pp. 251–266; Richard B. Davis, "The Principlism Debate: A Critical Overview," *The Journal of Medicine and Philosophy*, 20 (1995): 85–105; K. Danner Clouser and Bernard Gert, "Concerning Principlism and Its Defenders: Reply to Beauchamp and Veatch," *Building Bioethics: Conversations with Clouser and Friends on Medical Ethics*, ed. Loretta M. Kopelman (Dordrecht: Kluwer Academic Publishers, 1999), pp. 183–199.

16. Raymond J. Devettere, "The Principled Approach: Principles, Rules, and Actions," *Meta Medical Ethics: The Philosophical Foundations of Bioethics*, ed. Michael A. Grodin (Dordrecht: Kluwer Academic Publishers, 1995), pp. 27–28, italics added.

17. John Stuart Mill, *Utilitarianism* (Buffalo: Prometheus Books, 1987, originally published 1863), p. 49.

18. Earl R. Winkler, "From Kantianism to Contextualism: The Rise and Fall of the Paradigm Theory in Bioethics," *Applied Ethics: A Reader*, eds. Earl R. Winkler and Jerrold R. Coombs (Oxford: Blackwell, 1993), p. 355. For different formulations of the objection, see Albert R. Jonsen, "Casuistry: An Alternative or Complement to Principles?" *Kennedy Institute of Ethics Journal*, 5 (1995): 237–251; Albert R. Jonsen and

Stephen Toulmin, *The Abuse of Casuistry* (Berkeley: University of California Press, 1988).

19. Childress, "A Principle-Based Approach," p. 68.

Five

THE METHOD OF WIDE REFLECTIVE EQUILIBRIUM IN BIOETHICS

Juha Räikkä

1. What Is Wide Reflective Equilibrium?

The method of wide reflective equilibrium has been widely applied in practical ethics and especially in bioethics. In what follows I would like to say few words on the nature of this method.

The method of wide reflective equilibrium (WRE) is a coherence method of justification in ethics. WRE was first introduced by John Rawls in his "The Independence of Moral Theory," and one of WRE's strongest proponents has been another American philosopher Norman Daniels.[1] As Daniels describes WRE, it is a method which attempts to produce coherence in an ordered triple of sets of beliefs held by a particular person, namely (a) a set of considered moral judgments, (b) a set of moral principles, and (c) a set of relevant (scientific and philosophical) background theories.[2]

When using WRE, a person begins by collecting moral judgments (such as "abortion should be allowed") which she finds intuitively plausible. Then she proposes alternative sets of moral principles (such as "killing human beings is wrong") that have varying degree of fit with the moral judgments. Finally, she seeks support for those moral judgments and moral principles from background theories (such as "a fetus is not a human being") that are, in her view, acceptable. As Daniels writes, we can imagine the agent working back and forth, making adjustments to her considered moral judgments, her moral principles and her background theories. Finally, she arrives at an equilibrium point that consists of the ordered triple (a), (b) and (c). Moral judgments included in this point are taken to be *justified*. Reaching such a point may be difficult; as Rawls puts it, achieving it is an ideal situation.

One may try to use WRE collectively, and in a sense, daily moral discussions are in fact guided by WRE (even if participants of such discussions have rarely heard about the method). When person S1 thinks that she is justified in accepting certain moral judgment a1, person S2 may point out that a1 is not consistent with the moral principle b1, which must be attractive also from S1's point of view. This is how normative and ethical discussions normally proceed.

However, it is important to keep in mind that WRE is a normative method—it tells how an ethical evaluation *should* proceed—and not merely a description of actual discussions.[3]

2. The Acceptability of WRE

WRE has raised many critical responses. For instance, critics have claimed that WRE is really a form of moral intuitionism. According to this line of criticism, WRE implies that a person is justified in believing whatever she happens to believe, if she has a strong enough "intuition" that this or that is so (for instance, that "abortion should be allowed"). This argument, however, seems unfounded. Intuitionist theories are usually foundationalist in a sense that "intuitions" or at least some of them are thought to be somehow incorrigible or basic or self–warranting. But WRE allows corrections of moral judgments: none of them are thought to be "basic," whatever the strength of one's intuition.[4]

Is WRE anything else than a clever way to systematize our moral judgments? According to the critics it is not, but defenders have argued that WRE is much more than that. In their view, background theories (c) give independent support to moral judgments and principles, and background theories may be justified independently of the fact that they cohere with attractive moral judgments and principles. The method of narrow reflective equilibrium (NRE) seeks coherence only between moral judgments and moral principles. But WRE is wider than NRE in that it takes background theories into account.

An obvious problem with WRE seems to be that the considered moral judgments (a) are not initially credible. Instead, they are a result of "accidents." Even sincerely believed and carefully formulated moral judgments may be biased by self–interest, self–deception, and cultural and historical influences.[5] This is problematic, since the ordered triple (a), (b) and (c) is partly justified by referring to the considered moral judgments. This problem is not the general problem of all coherence accounts of justification, but a particularly serious problem faced by WRE.[6]

According to Daniels, however, the "no credibility" objection is merely a burden–of–proof argument.[7] He writes that it is "plausible to think that only the development of acceptable moral theory in wide reflective equilibrium will enable us to determine what kind of 'fact,' if any, is involved in a considered moral judgment." While we have to confess that some answer to the question about the reliability of moral judgments is required, there is no reason to think that there is no such answer. Hence we are justified in using WRE and trusting in its results.

Does WRE open doors to moral relativism? Is it not likely that eventually there will be not only one equilibrium point shared by all or most people, but various different equilibrium points? If so, we will also have different answers to ethical questions (such as "should abortion be allowed?") all of which will be equally justified.[8] This worry was raised already by Rawls, and there is no easy way to answer it. We should keep in mind, however, that seeking WRE may be an endless process, and we can always challenge each other's beliefs of establishing such an equilibrium point. Another important issue is that WRE may assist in producing greater moral agreement, since the method uses background theories and may thus render problems more tractable.[9]

3. Concluding Remarks

WRE is not explicitly connected to particular views on moral ontology or the nature of moral truths. A proponent of WRE may think that it will lead us to moral truths or closer to moral truths if there are any. But the constraints WRE puts on the acceptability of moral judgments are coherence constraints, which are not related to claims of truth as such.[10]

WRE has been widely applied in practical ethics and social philosophy. Too often these applications have been based on the false hope that the explicit use of WRE adds something important to the arguments that are presented in the discussion in any case. It does not, although it may be pleasant and valuable to be aware of the method one is using.

Suppose that I am criticizing your view that homosexual couples are not entitled to a right to adopt a child. My argument is that parents' sex is not relevant to child's well being. Obviously, I am using WRE here, but the argument will not become any better if I explicitly point out that here I am "working back and forth," trying to find a consistent equilibrium point that we both should accept. My argument is good or bad regardless of my knowledge or ignorance of the methodological issues.

NOTES

1. John Rawls, *A Theory of Justice* (Oxford: Clarendon Press, 1972); John Rawls, "The Independence of Moral Theory" (1975), reprinted in John Rawls, *Collected Papers* (Harvard University Press, Cambridge 1999), pp. 286–302.
   2. Norman Daniels, *Justice and Justification* (Cambridge: Cambridge University Press, 1996), p. 22.
   3. *Cf.* Bo Petersson, (ed.), *Applied Ethics and Reflective Equilibrium* (Linköping: Centre for Applied Ethics, 2000), p. 29.
   4. *Cf.* Roger P. Ebertz, "Is Reflective Equilibrium a Coherentist Model?" *Canadian Journal of Philosophy*, 23 (1987), pp. 193–214.
   5. Juha Räikkä, "Are There Alternative Methods in Ethics?" *Grazer Philosophische Studien*, 52 (1996), pp. 173–189.
   6. *Cf.* Michael DePaul, "Two Conceptions of Coherence Methods in Ethics", *Mind*, 96 (1987), pp. 463–481.

7. Daniels, *Justice and Justification*, p. 31.

8. Fred D'Agostino, "Relativism and Reflective Equilibrium", *The Monist*, 71 (1988), pp. 420–436.

9. *Cf.* Wibren van der Burg and Theo van Willigenburg, (eds.), *Reflective Equilibrium* (Dordrecht: Kluwer, 1998).

10. *Cf.* Margaret Holmgren, "Wide Reflective Equilibrium and Objective Moral Truth", *Metaphilosophy*, 18 (1987), pp. 108–124.

Six

BUT HOW COULD THEY KNOW? REFLECTIONS ON THE ROLE OF PHILOSOPHY AND PHILOSOPHERS IN MEDICAL ETHICS

Pekka Louhiala

1. Introduction

"They say you really become a doctor after you've killed a few patients." With these words a young resident comforted an intern who had just lost a patient. This scene took place in the television show *ER*.

I do not know what lay people thought when they saw this particular episode of *ER,* but I guess that I am not the only physician who immediately felt that this short sentence caught something very essential about being a physician, or more precisely, *becoming* a physician.

"But how could they know? They've never been there in the middle of the night, helplessly watching a patient die and wondering painfully what could have saved her life." These were the words of a colleague when we were discussing the role philosophers could have in medical ethics.

Philosophers certainly have had a role in medical ethics since the 1960s, when modern bioethics was introduced. But what kind of role should philosophy and philosophers have then? It depends, first, upon the view we have of philosophy.

2. Narrow and Broad Views of Philosophy

"Philosophy is not only useless, but also dangerous. Philosophy has produced nothing else but a cemetery of theoretical systems; but these dead systems are haunting us like ghosts. Half of the philosophers are engaged in trying to kill these ghosts again and again; the other half is busy to revive the same ghosts. The best strategy is to ignore philosophy and to separate it as strongly as possible from medicine." These are the thoughts of the German psychiatrist E. Bleuler, who summarized his opinion in the following aphorism: "Philosophy is fine and science is fine, but combined they are like a mixture of garlic and chocolate."[1]

Obviously, many physicians and researchers in medicine share Bleuler's thoughts today and think that there should be no place for philosophy in the medical curriculum, for example. It is as obvious that Bleuler's and his modern followers' opinion refers to a rather narrow view of philosophy.

There are, however, many broader views of philosophy, although the definition or the nature of philosophy pose questions on which philosophers typically disagree.

The Oxford Companion to Philosophy opens the entry "philosophy" by describing first the difficulty: "Most definitions of philosophy are fairly controversial, particularly if they aim to be at all interesting or profound."[2] A short definition or characterization is, however, given later: "Philosophy is thinking about thinking." Martyn Evans, a British philosopher of medicine, has said the same thing in other words: "philosophy of medicine asks questions about the questions medicine asks." If philosophy is understood this way, medicine—or any other human activity!—immediately offers a multitude of questions to which the answer cannot be found *within* the activity. "Is Mr. Brown healthy?" is a medical question ("first order question") but "What is health?" is a question that cannot be answered without reference to something outside medicine ("second order question").

Another broad characterization of philosophy is offered by D. D. Raphael, a British moral philosopher: "the main purpose of philosophy, as practiced in the Western tradition, is the critical evaluation of assumptions and arguments."[3] Applying this idea to medicine and medical ethics means simply that evaluating the multitude of moral issues related to the science and practice of medicine is a *philosophical* task.

3. Whose Business Is Medical Ethics?

For a long time, the medical profession thought that medical ethics belonged to it and it only. The academic world or the public did not disagree to a great extent. In the late 1960s, however, the climate changed, and, first, some Catholic theologians, then philosophers, became more and more interested and involved in medical ethics. There were many reasons for this transition: the rapid technological development in medicine after the Second World War; the rise of individualism in general and women's and children's rights movement in particular; the Vietnam war and its impact on the political activity of philosophers. In addition, the inability of biomedicine to solve all the major health problems of the world had become obvious. First, medical ethics, and later more generally the philosophy of medicine, were called upon to help resolve the identity crisis of medicine.

The involvement of philosophers and philosophy in medicine grew rapidly during the 1970s and 1980s, and the disciplines of philosophical medical ethics, bioethics and clinical ethics were established. The representatives of the latter offered consultations in ethical problems in the same way that specialists in medical sub-disciplines consult in their own areas of expertise.

Philosophers do not agree on many things. Is it realistic, then, to expect that they can contribute in a meaningful way to solving the very practical problems of medical ethics in real life?

If a simple answer is expected, it is, no, they cannot contribute. Expertise in moral philosophy does not provide the expertise in the moral dilemmas of medicine needed in order that a philosopher can say what is right or wrong in a particular situation. Philosophical medical ethics is not like engineering. When concrete, real-life dilemmas are faced, philosophers, physicians, nurses and lay people are all on the same level: no one has more expertise than anyone else. Or, as one of my students suggested, if someone has, it must be the patient. Patients are the main actors, and the practice and science of medicine would not exist without their problems and suffering.

Philosophy and philosophers can, however, contribute to medical ethics in other important ways. Because medicine is so deeply a value-laden discipline, philosophers have a lot of work in merely exploring the values in various medical settings. Conceptual analysis is one of the tools of philosophers. Medicine, if any discipline, is full of vague concepts. Both philosophy and medicine can gain from this co-operation: philosophical problems in medicine provide a real challenge to philosophy, which can, in turn, help clarify the discussion within medicine.

4. Expertise in Medical Ethics

What is the nature of expertise in medical ethics? Does it differ from, for example, expertise in medicine or some of its subdisciplines?

To see the similarities and differences, we have to look at what the experts in each field do and know. A nephrologist, for example, has special knowledge on the functions and diseases of the kidneys. Although any decision in medicine is based on both facts and values, the content of a nephrologist's judgments is primarily factual. With respect to this factual content, he is superior to the physician asking for the consultation. In most cases the consultant and the patient agree about the value judgments and the nephrologist is consulted because of his expertise in the facts.

In the case of an ethical dilemma, however, the primary disagreement concerns values. A medical ethicist has special knowledge about ethical theory and the exploration of values. There is, however, a distinction between knowing a lot about ethical theory and knowing what the morally right thing to do is in this particular situation.

What is it, then, that characterizes the position of the medical ethicist? Philosophical training has probably increased the ethicist's ability to discern a wider range of potentially relevant factors in ethically complex cases than the physician would ordinarily be able to discern. With this ability the ethicist can certainly contribute to the case, but, even with this ability he or she has not gained authority over anyone else involved in the case. In fact, training in philosophy could also affect the moral sensitivity of a person, but, again, this person cannot claim to have any authority over others in particular cases.

Even among the supporters of so-called clinical ethics, there is disagreement about who should (or could) practice it. Philosopher David Thomasma, one of the pioneers, argued very strongly that philosophers can and even ought to offer ethics consultations.[4] In contrast, physician-ethicists Siegler, Pellegrino and Singer have argued equally strongly that only people trained in medicine are capable of working properly as clinical ethics consultants since they "enjoy the advantages of a firm grasp of the factual tripod upon which ethical decisions must rest: diagnosis, prognosis and therapy."[5]

5. Philosophical Medical Ethics

Sociologists can be considered the predecessors of philosophers in interdisciplinary endeavors with medicine, and the role of medical sociology provides an analogy that may clarify the status of medical ethics.[6] If sociology unquestioningly accepts the medical definition of the "problem," it loses the critical distance, which, on the other hand, may prove fruitful for medicine in general. In the same way, it is important that medical ethics is able to keep the distance necessary for some practices to be examined critically. As Barnard put it: "ethics and humanities must ask to what extent their desire for acceptance in the clinic requires their acceptance of the clinic."[7]

Whatever the solution of an ethical problem is, it is health care professionals who must do the practical work. Therefore, their views are of special importance when compared with those of outsiders. Philosopher Carl Elliot has demonstrated this role of health care professionals brilliantly in his paper "Philosopher-Assisted Suicide and Euthanasia,"[8] in which he—obviously as a thought experiment—suggests that philosophers are trained to assist in suicides. The simple justification is that many philosophers have very actively argumented for active euthanasia, while most physicians (excluding the Netherlands) are against it. The basic message of Elliot seems to be that the views of those who have to put the decisions into practice are, after all, highly relevant.

It may be wise and clarifying to add the attribute *philosophical* to medical ethics when one refers to the work philosophers do. In his thesis, Matti Häyry examined the nature of applied philosophy in general and medical ethics in particular.[9] Abstract philosophy cannot be directly applied by deriving practical norms from agreed general moral laws. This "engineering model" should be abandoned but it does not mean that philosophy is useless.

According to Häyry, the first task of applied philosophy—in medicine and elsewhere—is to uncover the principles and codes recognized in the social environment that is studied.[10] The second task is rational reconstruction that aims at "spelling out moral rules, norms and principles which, taken as a whole, would fulfill the conditions of consistency and rational acceptability, as defined by the deep metaphysical assumptions prevailing in the examined community."[11]

It is easy to agree about the first task, which also sounds realistic. It may, however, be unrealistic to expect that the second task, rational reconstruction, can be fully completed when serious moral dilemmas are at stake.

6. Conclusion

"But how could they know?" asked my friend. How do I respond? Certainly they cannot "know" but neither can we physicians, although we often think that we can. Medical education and expertise do not give us superiority when it comes to value judgments, neither does philosophical education and expertise give authority in moral issues. Philosophy and philosophers can, however, contribute in many meaningful and fruitful ways to medical ethics. We in the medical community should be humble enough to recognize that. And philosophers should be humble enough to recognize that having to carry out the practical consequences of moral judgments matters.

ACKNOWLEDGEMENTS

I thank Veikko Launis, Raimo Puustinen, and Simo Vehmas for comments.

NOTES

1. E. Bleuler, *Naturgeschichte der Seele und ihres Bewusztwerdens: Eine Elementarpsychologie* (Berlin: Springer, 1921) cited in Henk ten Have, "Medical Philosophy and the Cultivation of Humanity," *Medicine, Health Care and Philosophy*, 2:1 (1999), pp. 1–2.

2. Ted Honderich (ed.), *The Oxford Companion to Philosophy* (Oxford: Oxford University Press, 1995), p. 666.

3. D. D. Raphael, *Moral Philosophy* (Oxford: Oxford University Press, 1994), p. 1.

4. David Thomasma, "Why Philosophers Should Offer Ethics Consultations," *Theoretical Medicine*, 12 (1991), pp. 129–140.

5. Mark Siegler, Edmund D. Pellegrino and Peter A. Singer, "Clinical Med cal Ethics," *The Journal of Clinical Ethics*, 1 (1990), pp. 5–9.

6. David Barnard, "Reflections of a Reluctant Clinical Ethicist: Ethics Consulta-tion and the Collapse of Critical Distance," *Theoretical Medicine*, 13 (1992), pp. 15–22.

7. Barnard, "Reflections of a Reluctant Clinical Ethicist."

8. Carl Elliott, "Philosopher Assisted Suicide and Euthanasia," *British Med cal Journal*, 313 (1996), pp. 1088–1089.

9. Matti Häyry, *Critical Studies in Philosophical Medical Ethics* (Helsinki: De-partment of Philosophy, University of Helsinki, 1990).

10. Häyry, *Critical Studies in Philosophical Medical Ethics*, p. 11.

11. Häyry, *Critical Studies in Philosophical Medical Ethics*, p. 13.

Seven

DOES NURSING ETHICS FIT IN WITH PHILOSOPHY AND BIOETHICS?

Leila Toiviainen

1. Nursing Ethics as a Distinct Discipline

The aim of this investigation is to show that nurses play a unique role in health care, and that nursing ethics is therefore a distinct field of study. While nurses must obviously build upon the foundations laid by traditional moral philosophy, nursing ethics as a discipline evolves from it—as does, for example, environmental ethics—as a distinct field of applied ethics with its own conceptual framework.

I have used the collection *Scratching the Surface of Bioethics*, edited by Matti Häyry and Tuija Takala, as the basis for my investigation into whether nursing ethics fits in with philosophy and bioethics. In that book, the authors emphasize the interdisciplinary nature of the bioethical endeavor; to this I want to add the voice of nursing, since it is silent in their deliberations.

I argue that nurses have particular skills not possessed by other health professionals, a fact which much philosophical or bioethical literature fails to recognize. We can trace the origin of these skills to the fact that nurses, unlike any other health professionals, provide round-the-clock care to patients in an almost unlimited variety of settings. The relationships they establish with patients and their families are more intimate and more demanding than the limited engagement typical of other health professionals. The involvement of nurses in the daily activities of dressing, feeding, and toileting patients confers a low status on the emerging profession in the eyes of some academics. However, I regard this intimate involvement in the daily lives of vulnerable individuals as a privilege, and one which confers upon nurses the right to speak for themselves on professional issues.

If nurses play an indispensable role in the health and wellbeing of their patients, then their ethics education must equip them for that role, providing them with the skills necessary for it. I explore the alternatives of who should provide them with this education and how it should be done. I do this from the perspective of a bioethics lecturer at the University of Tasmania and of a registered nurse working at a Tasmanian nursing home.

2. The Ethical Work of Nursing

Nurses deal with what Michael Parker terms "the kind of philosophical questions so intimately part of the human condition, like those of birth, death, love, and loss"[1] in a way that other health professionals do not. They are present not only momentarily but continuously. In the case of birth, they support families through the antenatal period, labor, delivery, postnatal, and home care. Nurses who work in neonatal intensive care look after premature babies on respirators; often those babies' lives end after weeks and months of improvements and deteriorations. The parents of these children obviously need ongoing support to prepare them for their loss.

At the other end of life, nurses working in nursing homes give residents care over months and years. During this time, they come not only to know the residents well, but also their families, and share in many of their joys and sorrows, such as the births of great-grandchildren or the loss of sons and daughters on the part of the oldest residents. Seriously ill residents sometimes confront nurses with euthanasia requests in the absence of doctors, or because the doctors are less approachable than nurses. As euthanasia is illegal in Australia, nurses must find ways of responding to the despair of individuals in place of and on behalf of doctors, while simultaneously acting within their scope of practice and within ethical guidelines. This is not an easy balancing act, but it is one of the unavoidable roles of a registered nurse.

In these situations nurses can, for instance, honestly state that they cannot perform acts of euthanasia, but that they can take nursing measures to allay the resident's anxiety, to assess the level of her physical and mental pain and distress, and to diagnose its causes and relay this information to the medical practitioner. First and foremost, nurses are the one permanent, reliable presence and comfort for patients and their families.

3. Nursing Ethics Education, Philosophy, and Bioethics

Students in schools of nursing in English speaking countries such as Australia, New Zealand, the United States, and the United Kingdom are taught ethics either by philosophers or nurses, or occasionally by nurse philosophers. If, as I argue, nurses have a special role in the provision of health care, then their education should reflect this. Nursing is a practical profession that demands a solid theoretical foundation on which nurses can base clinical judgements and practical actions that they can stand accountable for in front of the general public, and increasingly in courts of law. Ethics education should ideally do this by fitting theory and practice together into a coherent whole. If this is the case, then those teaching nurses need to know about the realities of their practice, while at the same time having a sound knowledge of moral philosophy and bioethics.

The sociologist Mairi Levitt claims that bioethicists do not ask empirical questions that have a direct bearing on everyday health care, for instance about the justification of a liver transplant for an ex-alcoholic who might take up drinking again and waste the donor liver.[2] Nurse ethicists certainly ask these questions. Douglas Olsen of Yale University School of Nursing, who previously worked as a community nurse in Alaska, has done empirical research to demonstrate that nurses find it more difficult to act ethically toward patients who in their judgement have caused their own problems, such as smokers, alcoholics, non-compliant diabetics, many AIDS victims, and patients who use violence and intimidation.[3] He also touches on economic and social issues, such as patients not being able to exercise freedom in choosing their health care provider, because they lack the knowledge necessary to do so.[4]

4. Nurses and Practical Moral Courage

In Australia we have in Toni Hoffman an example of a registered nurse who can combine ethical theory with nursing practice in a way that has led to legal action against a surgeon and hospital Management. She works in an intensive care unit at the Bundaberg Base Hospital in Queensland, where she reported the incompetent practices of a surgeon, Jayat Patel. Patel's practices had led to the deaths of several patients. Prior to this appointment she had worked for five years (including the Gulf War period) in Saudi Arabia with "a lot of really brilliant surgeons."[5] At the end of 2002 she completed her Master of Bioethics degree. Dr Patel started at Bundaberg Base Hospital in 2003. It has taken until this year for the matter to attract enough publicity for an investigation to be started into Dr. Patel's malpractice, and into the deaths of several of his patients.

Although one of the anesthetists had called Dr. Patel "Dr. Death," and had maintained that he would not want to be operated on by such a surgeon, and despite Dr Patel's colleagues being aware of his incompetence, he was not stopped from harming his patients. As a journalist reports, "There were doctors aware of what was going on, but they didn't respond as forcefully as the nurses, and in particular, Toni Hoffman."[6] The senior nurses in administration did not take her complaint seriously, but the Director of Nursing, Linda Mulligan "gave me a book to read on how to deal with difficult people. It wasn't that we were dealing with clinical incompetence and we needed someone to pay attention and listen."[7]

Although the case of Toni Hoffman as a whistle-blower on a surgeon who made numerous fatal mistakes is fortunately extreme, it highlights my argument that nursing ethics plays a role that is not only subsidiary to philosophy or bioethics, but extends to the very foundations of clinical practice. While nurses must understand the basics of deontology, it is hard to imagine that Kant could have provided Toni with adequate guidelines on how to act in this situation. And yet, Kant would have advised her to speak the truth without considering the consequences to herself, because of her duty to her patients. He would have failed, however, to appreciate the emotionally draining effects on Toni of dealing with distressed patients and relatives, and of her being bullied by the hospital Management and later the courts. She was, for instance, criticized failing to bring the matter to the attention of Management earlier.[8]

Toni Hoffman has been left to deal with the consequences of her truth telling. Her duty to her patients is fulfilled, but her life and career are on hold:

> I mean, we've been bullied and intimidated for so long now that I have no idea what the future holds. I probably have made some enemies because of this, but I did have to be a patient advocate. I think that I'll just keep going to work and I'll probably have some time off at the end of the year and go overseas and, I don't know, I don't know. I can't … I have no idea. Um … just get some normality back in my life. That would be good, I think.[9]

To be a nurse like Toni Hoffman, or even to be a part-time aged care nurse faced with euthanasia requests, requires the kind of practical moral courage not required of ordinary academic philosophers or bioethicists. They may limit their discussion of Toni Hoffman's dilemma to the consideration of arguments for and against abstract moral duties in the situation. They do not have to deal with powerful enemies in their workplace on a daily basis; unfortunately this is true of many nurses practicing in Australian public hospitals today.

5. Nursing as a Profession with Its Own Ethics

There is an argument levelled against nursing ethics as a discipline: if nursing is not a profession, how can nursing ethics be a discipline? Matti Häyry sets out the criteria for true professionals as outlined by, for instance, Ruth Chadwick:

- Specialized knowledge
- Long and intensive academic studies
- Permanent careers
- Organization and self-rule within the group
- As a group, a decisive role in the arrangement of the relevant studies, and in the recruitment of new members to the group
- A distinctive professional ethos, or morality within the work; and positions of considerable responsibility in communities and societies.[10]

Nurses, although acting on the instructions of a doctor, still need specialized knowledge of their own to carry out the orders. Many older persons in the nursing home where I work, for instance, need their medications crushed and mixed in pureed food. The nurse needs to know which drugs can be crushed and which capsules can be opened, and also to know which individuals can swallow whole tablets and which cannot. This is only possible if the nurse undertakes a swallowing assessment of the resident. She or he also needs to understand the ethical issues that pertain to the use of chemical restraints, and issues concerning deception and lack of informed consent. She or he also needs an awareness of the complex ethical and legal issues related to caring for people who are no longer competent to make decisions about their own care. It could be claimed that all of the above information is the field of other disciplines such a pharmacology, applied moral philosophy, or law. Nursing knowledge arises from these, however, in the theories and practice of the expert nurse who can synthesize all of the above information into a coherent whole that benefits the resident.

As the example of Toni Hoffman shows, nurses undertake long and intensive academic studies. The same cannot always be said of medical practitioners whose continuing education programs accredited by the Royal Australian College of General Practitioners include movie screenings and a "wealth creation" seminar that teaches GPs about investments, how to maximize their profits and even hide their assets from patients who may try to sue them. In the words of a South Australian GP James Moxham who finds the programs ethically unacceptable:

> It's possible to get all your points by going to drug-company-funded dinners, and you can fall asleep before the main speaker and you will still get your points.[11]

Australian general practitioners need to earn 130 continuing education points every three years; the wealth seminar was allocated 30 points and the movie screening six points. Registered nurses in Australia must be in possession of an annual practicing certificate; in order to be given this by a state nursing board they must sign a statutory declaration to say that they are practicing in their profession and adhere to the relevant legislation and ethical codes.

Although not all people who train in nursing make it their permanent career, most of my present colleagues are women who have practiced nursing for over 30 years in several countries and numerous settings in community and institutional care.

Nurses are members of professional organizations and colleges of nursing. Many of them are also members of the International Council of Nurses, which holds biennial conferences. This year's conference in Taipei had over 3000 delegates from over 100 countries. The International Centre for Nursing

Ethics at Surrey University offers ethics courses for nurses from all parts of the world. The Centre gives human rights awards for nurses who have distinguished themselves in their work.

6. The Future of Nursing Ethics

If nursing ethics is to serve the most vulnerable individuals, who most need those with moral courage to speak on their behalf, then it must include a global, political dimension. For this to become a reality, more and better-educated nurses supported by organizations such as the International Centre for Nursing Ethics and the International Council for Nurses are required to develop and articulate the unique position of nursing in health care in all countries and settings. In small part conference papers and book chapters such as this strive to put nursing ethics on the horizon of bioethics and philosophy as a distinct ethos of a profession with its own morality.

NOTES

1. Michael Parker, "Foreword," *Scratching the Surface of Bioethics*, eds. Matti Häyry and Tuija Takala, (Amsterdam: Rodopi) 2003, p. ix.
2. Mairi Levitt, "Better Together? Sociological and Philosophical Perspectives on Bioethics," *Scratching the Surface of Bioethics*, pp. 20–21.
3. Douglas Olsen, "When the Patient Causes the Problem: The Effect of Patient Responsibility on the Nurse-Patient Relationship," *Journal of Advanced Nursing*, 26 (1997), p. 518.
4. Douglas Olsen, "Provider Choice: Essential to Autonomy of Advertising Gimmick?" *Nursing Ethics*, 3:2 (1996), pp. 108–117.
5. Australian Broadcasting Corporation, *Australian Story: At Death's Door—Transcript*. Program Transcript Monday, 27th June, 2005.
6. Hedley Thomas, journalist *The Courier Mail*, in Australian Broadcasting Corporation, *Australian Story: At Death's Door—Transcript*. Program Transcript Monday, 27th June, 2005.
7. Toni Hoffman in *Australian Story: At Death's Door—Transcript*. Program Transcript Monday, 27th June, 2005.
8. Sean Parnell, "Scramble to Plug Dr Death Leaks," *The Weekend Australian Inquirer*, July 16–17, 2005, p. 30.
9. Toni Hoffman's concluding words in *Australian Story: At Death's Door—Transcript*. Program Transcript Monday, 27th June, 2005.
10. Matti Häyry, "Do Bioscientists Need Professional Ethics?" *Scratching the Surface of Bioethics*, eds. Matti Häyry and Tuija Takala, (Amsterdam: Rodopi, 2003), p. 92.
11. Adam Cresswell, "Doctors' Orders: Learn to Get Rich," *The Weekend Australian*, September 10–11, 2005, p. 3.

Part Three

DIGNITY, PRECAUTION, AND SOLIDARITY

Eight

DIGNITY: YET ANOTHER LOOK

Simon Woods

> So many roads, so much at stake
> So many dead ends, I'm at the edge of the lake
> Sometimes I wonder what it's gonna take
> To find dignity.[1]

1. Introduction

If only Bob Dylan had had the opportunity to read Ruth Macklin's[2] dismissal of dignity then perhaps he might have realized that his song-writing skills could have been put to better use! However I suspect that Dylan, like myself, would not be content to dismiss dignity as a mere "slogan." In this paper I will revisit the debate on the value of dignity to medical ethics by outlining Macklin's criticisms; posing some concerns about those criticisms; and finally offering an argument as to why dumping dignity is not the sort of economy of language that medical ethics needs. En route to this conclusion I shall refer to Matti Häyry's more moderate further look at dignity.[3] Whilst I agree with both Macklin and Häyry that dignity is sometimes used merely as a slogan, I conclude that this is not a reason to abandon it. Whilst dignity-as-slogan cases are relatively easy to find, they are not illustrative of instances of dignity in the context of medical ethics proper, and I shall turn to examples of these in order to discuss a more substantive version of dignity in the context of clinical medical ethics.

2. Macklin's Argument

Ruth Macklin writing in the *British Medical Journal* tells us "dignity is a useless concept."[4] Although references to dignity abound in contemporary ethics parlance, and more specifically it is claimed that certain developments in the medical sciences threaten to violate human dignity.

> A close inspection of leading examples shows that appeals to dignity
> are either vague restatements of other, more precise notions or mere

slogans that add nothing to the understanding of the topic … Dignity
is a useless concept in medical ethics and can be eliminated without
any loss of content[5]

There are three stands to Macklin's argument against dignity:

- Dignity is no more than a slogan.
- Dignity is vague.
- Dignity can be replaced by more precise terms.

I shall respond to these in turn.

Häyry comments that the contemporary use of "dignity" is legal or semi-
legal, and can be found in the constitutions of several modern nation states
before it was actively recruited to bolster the United Nations' *Universal Declaration of Human Rights* (1948) and sundry other declarations and statements
such as the Conseil de l'Europe *Convention for the Protection of Human
Rights and Dignity of the Human Being with regard to the Application of Biology and Medicine* (1997). Macklin's view is in agreement with this analysis as
she comments that this latter convention's use of "dignity" has no meaning
that cannot be exhausted by the principles of medical ethics. These she goes on
to unpack as "respect for persons," the need for voluntary informed consent,
protection of confidentiality, and the avoidance of discrimination and abusive
practices. Perhaps the point being made by Macklin is that "dignity" is used in
the examples cited above as if it were a technical term in ethics; for example
like "autonomy." However this appears to be rather a weak criticism since
many complex concepts are used in ways which imply that their meaning is
unambiguous, including "autonomy" itself. I suggest that medical ethics
should be engaged with unpacking concepts such as dignity, because if nothing
else it enables an exploration of some of those subtleties that medical ethics
requires.

However, Macklin's point is that dignity is useless in specifically *medical*
ethics, but she appeals to very few instances where this case can be made. One
example Macklin does give is the association of dignity with end of life decisions. Commenting upon the California Natural Death Act (1992), which recognizes the right of individuals to refuse life prolonging treatment, she comments that "dignity seems to be nothing other than respect for autonomy."
Macklin goes on to point out that the very notion of "death with dignity" has
been claimed by both advocates and opponents of euthanasia: "Dignitas" being
the name of the Swiss assisted suicide group whose maxim "live with dignity,
die with dignity" could equally be claimed by pro-life groups and the advocates of palliative care who are antithetical to assisted dying.[6] However the
pivotal use of a concept in opposing arguments is not unique to dignity.
Autonomy, a concept which Macklin believes to be a clearer and more precise

concept than dignity, is also used in a similar way; indeed respect for autonomy is specifically used both in support of assisted dying and against. Arguments using the principle of respect for autonomy are often used to support the right of a person to control the manner and timing of their own death as a claim about their right to self-determination. Autonomy arguments are also used against such a right, sometimes because it is said to infringe upon the autonomy of the person required to do the assisting. In addition, it is sometimes also argued that to insist that respect for autonomy requires that people be allowed to end their life with assistance is to misconstrue the scope of the principle of respect for autonomy: to use Daniel Callahan's words this is "self-determination run amok."[7] Therefore equal claim to competing interpretations of a concept is not a feature that is unique to dignity.

Macklin also comments upon the concerns expressed about dignity in the context of managing human corpses in the medical context, in particular the use of the newly dead by medical students to practice clinical procedures. Reflecting upon the charge made by some medical ethicists that this is a violation of dignity, Macklin responds by pointing out that since the dead are no longer *autonomous* then this concern is misplaced. Macklin makes this move because she seems to believe that concerns about the deceased expressed in terms of dignity are in reality concerns about autonomy, and since the dead have no autonomy they ergo have no dignity to be violated; but this really avoids the issue of dignity by diverting the point to a discussion of autonomy. Macklin does however acknowledge that there may be reasonable enough concern for the sentiments of the deceased person's relatives to refrain from such practices out of respect for those wishes.

However the claim that concerns regarding the deceased person's dignity can be reduced to concerns for the wishes of the deceased's relatives is itself problematic. This is where there is pressure on Macklin to explain what she means by respect for autonomy and what specific implications it has in these contexts. Presumably the wishes of relatives are not worthy of respect merely because they are their wishes, but because the reason or reasons underpinning their wishes are regarded as valid and a convincing ground that their request be respected? The wishes alone are not sufficient, it is rather the reasons in which the wishes are grounded which renders them sufficient or not. I am against the reductionist turn in bioethics which sees ethical justification in terms of the lowest common denominator: we should rather attempt to do justice to the complexity of situations. For the surviving family, the corpse of the recently deceased may not, in their minds, be entirely separated from the person whom the corpse once was. For most people it is the grieving process which allows for this separation between corpse and person to take place, but in the immediate aftermath of death it seems reasonable to treat the corpse as if it were the person. In regarding the corpse as the person then it would seem justified to respect the corpse in a way that the living person would have expected to be treated with regard to their bodily integrity, modesty and respect.

Macklin's approach here is typical of many bio-ethicists who can be accused of representing the issues as overly black and white, so as to simplify in their own favor.[8] The question of whether, with regard to dignity, there is a right or wrong way to treat a corpse is not solely a matter of individual preferences. There is hardly a human culture that does not have deeply held beliefs, often expressed in ritual, about the respect owed to the human corpse.[9] Nor is it beyond reason to suggest that such beliefs might be the basis of laws, which may dictate more precise boundaries as to what is and is not permissible, as Nussbaum argues: "we humans need law precisely because we are vulnerable to harm and damage in many ways."[10] Of course the objections of the bereaved may not be grounded in a belief any deeper than the thought that "Granny was such a private person she would be dreadfully embarrassed to be used in that way," but as an expression of a concern regarding dignity this seems clear enough. It is not difficult to imagine several other scenarios in which relatives object to the particular uses of their deceased loved one's cadaver for training medical students. This is not to say that an argument could not be made for adopting alternative approaches to the dead, particularly where it could be argued that such changes might render some concrete benefit to the quick, but however good the argument it is unlikely to be sufficient justification for imposing such a change without a process of broad social accommodation and adjustment. However, the question of whether it is ever right to override the wishes of the living or the dead is a related and important question but a digression from the matter at hand.

3. Dignity and Human Genetics

A further area commented upon by both Macklin and Häyry is the application of the concept in the context of human genetics and reproductive research. Häyry points to what he considers the "most perplexing dignity-based document," UNESCO's *Universal declaration on the Human Genome and Human Rights*, which he summarizes as arguing that every bearer of human genes is also a bearer of human dignity with a right to be respected as such. Respect for dignity, amongst other things, precludes reproductive cloning.[11] Macklin also comments upon the US President's Council on Bioethics first report *Human Cloning and Human Dignity*[12] which gives a prominent place to the concept of dignity. The report states that "a begotten child comes into the world just as its parents once did, and is therefore their equal in dignity and humanity."[13] Because the report contains no analysis of dignity or how it relates to ethical principles such as respect for persons and provides no criteria for the violation of dignity then the concept "remains hopelessly vague." Although there are many well worked through arguments against human reproductive cloning,[14] to invoke the concept of dignity without clarifying its meaning in some detail in this context is, as Macklin suggests, to use a mere slogan. However the observation that a term is used as a slogan does not preclude the possibility that an effective slogan draws upon established meaning. In this context, the wrongness of cloning may imply the wrongful instrumental use of a human being, an argument that is consistent with a Kantian view of dignity.[15]

Macklin notes that one bioethics group that has gone someway towards defining human dignity is the Nuffield Council on Bioethics.[16] This report goes well beyond the US President's Council in specifying a meaning of dignity in research on behavioral genetics. The report refers to the sense of responsibility as "an essential ingredient in the conception of human dignity, in the presumption that one is a person whose actions, thoughts and concerns are worthy of intrinsic respect, because they have been chosen, organized and guided in a way which makes sense from a distinctively individual point of view."[17] Macklin argues that although this renders the concept of human dignity meaningful, it is nothing more than a capacity for rational thought and action, the central features conveyed in the principle of respect for autonomy. In this specific context, I am inclined to agree with Macklin and Häyry that attempts to equate human dignity with some form of genetic essentialism is misplaced and highly problematic.

Why, then, do so many articles and reports appeal to human dignity, as if it means something over and above respect for persons or for their autonomy? A possible explanation as Häyry suggests are the many religious sources that refer to human dignity, especially but not exclusively in Roman Catholic writings.[18] However, religious sources cannot explain how and why dignity has crept into the secular literature in medical ethics.

Of course the heritage of "dignity" is an ancient one and by reflecting on these pre-Christian sources as well as more contemporary ethical themes I will suggest how claims about dignity may be distinguished from claims about the respect for persons and autonomy.

4. Dignity: A Brief History

Both Macklin and Häyry's accounts of dignity are relatively contemporary; both also express puzzlement as to why the term should have entered contemporary bioethics. Dignity has a much longer history, and by reflecting on this longer history I shall suggest that there is a relatively robust contemporary meaning which is also consistent with its long historical tradition. Dignity or "Dignitas" takes its place as one of the classical virtues alongside others such as gravitas and humanitas: such virtues were regarded as intrinsic, for example to the Via Romana, the Roman way of life.[19] Dignity in this context has the meaning of a sense of self-worth and personal pride. Whilst I accept that there may be quite specific cultural and historical perspectives on what sustains or diminishes dignity, the idea that dignity is associated with esteem is consistent. Contingencies aside, the abiding sense of the meaning of dignity as a condition of personal value which contributes to an individual's self-image and self-worth is a central component of dignity and one which has contemporary resonance.

The history of dignity can be seen in examples of humanity's reflection on what it is to be essentially human, expressed through art and literature. The many forms of human representation and self-representations in art, in philosophical thought, and in personal reflection are rich sources for our purpose. The classical writer Cicero applies the term "dignity" to the human race, as that quality which distinguishes humans from animals:

> But in every investigation into the nature of duty, it is vitally necessary for us to remember always how vastly superior is man's nature to that of cattle and other animals their only thought is for bodily satisfactions .... Man's mind on the contrary, is developed by study and reflection .... [20]

The dignity of humanity has often been expressed in terms of the status of humanity over animals and with the association of humanity with God, a familiar theme within the Judeo-Christian tradition, for example, as expressed in Genesis 1:26, "And God said, Let us make man in our image, after our likeness ...."

These reflections upon mankind's status vis a vis that of other animals, and the association of the human with the divine, are common enough examples of human self-aggrandisement. Common themes in both Classical and Christian art and literature attempt to express the esteem of humans in terms of quality of mind and body. This combination of the classical and the Christian is reflected in Hamlet's famous speech that is arguably the epitome of the Renaissance self-reflexive individual:

> What a piece of work is man! How noble in reason! How infinite in faculties! In form and moving, how express and admirable! In action how like an angel! In apprehension, how like a god! The beauty of the world! The paragon of animals! And yet, to me, what is this quintessence of dust?[21]

The idea of being divine or god-like is but one common convention in humanity's exploration of human dignity, and what these examples show is that reflecting upon the status of humanity is an abiding preoccupation of people, a part of man's reflexivity. Hobbes, by contrast, notes quite different social conventions associated with dignity when he comments that:

> The value, or worth of a man, is as of all other things, his price; that is to say, so much as would be given for the use of his power: and therefore

not absolute; but a thing dependent on the need and judgement of another
... And as in other things, so in men, not the seller, but the buyer determines the Price. For let a man (as most men do) rate themselves as the
highest value they can; yet their true value is no more than it is esteemed
by others.[22]

Hobbes is right in his observation that there are such social conventions associated with dignity, but wrong to suggest that such conventions are indicative
of how dignity ought to be construed morally speaking. Clearly Hobbes is no
sophisticated psychologist, but I would suggest that from our brief dip into the
history of ideas two aspects of dignity are significant. The first is the aspect of
dignity associated with status as reflected in the regard given to the body. The
second is the internalized value the individual gives to him or herself, external
or objective esteem and self-esteem. To understand the ethical implications of
dignity we need to separate the social conventions from the morally substantive aspects. This requires us to understand the particular wrong done when
dignity is given no regard, and this arises in the many circumstances in which a
human being is treated in ways in which they ought not to be treated. This is
not something to be discovered a priori, although there has been an abiding
tradition of such attempts. We do however have many *a posteriori* exemplars
in human history which go some way to giving such an account. The Holocaust has perhaps provided some of the most profoundly disturbing examples
of institutionalized machinery bent on destroying human dignity. The Holocaust also provides some of the most profoundly inspiring examples of how
the spark of human dignity may survive, despite such insults. Primo Levi, a
survivor of the concentration camps, describes the phenomenon of the "musselmänner," slang for those individuals who had been rendered prostrate,
crushed by the lager (camp) machinery:

All the musselmans who finished in the gas chambers have the same
story, or more exactly, have no story; they followed the slope down to the
bottom, like the streams that run down to the sea. On their entry into the
camp, through basic incapacity, or by misfortune, or through some banal
incident, they are overcome before they can adapt themselves; they are
beaten by time, they do not begin to learn German, to disentangle the in-
fernal knot of laws and prohibitions until their body is already in decay,
and nothing can save them from selections or from death by exhaustion.
Their life is short, but their number is endless: they, the Musselmänner, ...
form the backbone of the camp, an anonymous mass, continually renewed and always identical, of non-men who march and labor in silence,
the divine spark dead within them, already too empty really to suffer....
[I]f I could enclose all the evil of our time in one image, I would choose
this image which is so familiar to me: an emaciated man, with head

dropped and shoulders curved, on whose face and in whose eyes not a trace of a thought is to be seen.[23]

Levi and other writers[24] have also given examples of how some individuals maintained a sense of dignity, and a related will to survive, even in the face of such a sustained onslaught as the Holocaust. These accounts of human tragedy and personal survivorship give an insight into aspects of human psychology that are relevant to dignity. How a person is treated either by other individuals or by institutions can have an impact on that person's dignity, both in terms of their objective esteem and in the sense of their own value or self-esteem: both are of moral import to medical ethics.

Turning now to contemporary issues of dignity and medical ethics, is there anything we can conclude from this brief account? The ethical issue of dignity is concerned with the question of how people ought to be treated. This has implications for the conventions and standards of professional practice including communication skills, conventions of decency and privacy and so on. Evaluation of these standards ought to be mindful of the potential impact of such behaviors on our ideas about the value of that person in general, and the particular impact on that individual in terms of how they value themselves. The relevance of dignity to medical ethics can be seen in terms of a general normative question: "how ought we to treat people"? But dignity requires particular regard to "bodily" treatment and also awareness of the impact of medical treatment and care upon the concept of self-esteem. It should be clear without argument that the first of these aspects of dignity is relevant to medical ethics, but *both* are indeed relevant and centrally important to ethical medical practice because both are linked.

To be in a position to judge a health worker's action as unethical then one must be able to articulate what it is they are responsible for, in order to judge that they have failed in what they could reasonably be expected to do, or refrain from doing. It is reasonable to expect health workers to have awareness of the impact of routine medical care and treatment on the patient's self-esteem, since this is related to the general duty to be mindful of a patient's welfare. The self-evaluative aspect of dignity is linked because a person's self-esteem can be influenced by their awareness of how they are valued as this is reflected through the attitudes and behaviors of others. A simple if prosaic example of this is captured in the possible positive or negative affect of a professional's "bed-side manner." However I will spell out these claims through a number of examples.

The impact that medicine has upon society generally and on patients in particular has been the subject of much conceptual debate and empirical research.[25] It has long been recognized that medicine as an institution has been and is a powerful force in society. Sociologists have described the phenomenon of medicalization[26] and many have been critical of the forms this has taken, including the critique of medicine's approach to mental health.[27] The nineteenth century witnessed a growing awareness of the abuse and exploitation of people contained within the asylums or "Madhouses." This awareness eventually resulted in legislation and regulation to establish appropriate standards of care and treatment. Recognition of the moral implications and social and psychological drawbacks of such places have led to more reforms and much study of the "institutions." Erving Goffman's coining of the phrase "total institution" was in the context of his documenting the indignities of institutionalized care.[28] Other critics have commented upon the use of power within the wider institution of medicine and health with emphasis upon the disempowering nature of being in the patient's role.[29] Still others have focused upon particular disease states and the way that medicine has failed to distinguish between the disease and the person with the disease.[30] Awareness of the stigmatizing affects of disease and medical processes is an important and necessary aspect of the moral awareness of health workers.

There has been a shift in medical ethics from medical *etiquette* to substantive medical ethics. This can be expressed in terms of the necessity not merely to identify in abstract terms the principles that apply in medical practice, but to be specific about the standards which characterize *good* practice. This has been recognized by the educators of health professionals and reflected in the numerous approaches adopted in the education process, both to draw attention to standards of practice, and to attempt to assess that the doctor or nurse in preparation has begun to grasp these and to incorporate them into their way of working. Couching these concerns in terms of impact on human dignity is a useful way of exploring these complex issues with health workers.

Dignity is a challenging concept and no doubt will remain so. One of the interesting puzzles is whether dignity can be bestowed or diminished, since as we have seen the extrinsic factors thought to enhance or diminish dignity do not have a uniform effect upon the self-evaluative dimension. According to Levi, some lager prisoners were able to maintain an inner core of dignity despite the worst that the lager could offer. Some people find the indignity of disease too much to bear despite acknowledging the kindness and good care provided by others. A friend in the advance stages of multiple sclerosis commented that "there is no dignity left when you have to rely upon others to assist with your bladder function and to empty your bowels." Why should we keep dignity given this damning indictment? My response is that one can begin to distinguish between the instantiation of principles within a practice, which sets the standard for that practice, the *normative* standard, from the range of complex ways in which a person's dignity may be affected. The disease process may be accompanied by all manner of indignities but the way a nurse or doctor cares for a patient in those circumstances can, if they behave insensitively, exacerbate the indignity, or if they behave sensitively and ethically, go a long way towards ameliorating those indignities. Sensitive ethical behavior includes

many skills, verbal skills, body language, and awareness of the potential for
the patient's distress to name but a few.

Let us be reminded that medical ethics is about the good that medicine
and health care aims at and how this is achieved. To understand the potential
that medicine has to benefit and do harm to people requires a careful empirical
analysis of the impact, not just of medical interventions but also of medical
practice as a whole. This includes not only analyses of the impact of medical
treatments and therapies, the methods of providing medical services, but also
analysis of the impact of the relationship between the health worker and the
patient.

5. Conclusion

In this brief paper I have attempted to show that that there is something of
moral substance associated with the concept of dignity that is both relevant to
medical ethics and worth preserving. There are aspects of dignity that are relative to time and place but then which meanings are not? Macklin herself rec-
ommends autonomy as a concept central to medical ethics yet one which is
diversely interpreted and is often regarded as only specifically relevant to an
Anglo-American cultural context. Macklin's dismissal of dignity is perfunc-
tory and hasty. Häyry's is by contrast both balanced and thoughtful. Häyry
may be critical of dignity as a slogan, but he suggests that by comparing and
disputing the meaning of dignity we may "further understanding between people and cultures."[31]

Dignity, understood in terms of objective esteem and self-esteem of the
patient, is important to medical ethics. The moral imperative for medicine is to
be aware of the impact of both disease and medical practice upon a patient's
dignity, and to act according to that awareness. Dignity may be vague but then
so are many other concepts, which are nevertheless regarded as important in
medical ethics.[32] This is partly because we are still in the process of unpacking
such concepts and in a socially complex and changing world we must endeavor to continue to do so.

NOTES

1. "Dignity." Words and Music by Bob Dylan, Special Rider Music, 1994.
2. Ruth Macklin, "Dignity is a Useless Concept," *British Medical Journal*, 327
(2003), pp. 1419–1420.
3. Matti Häyry, "Another Look at Dignity," *Cambridge Quarterly of Healthcare
Ethics*, 13 (2004), pp. 7–14
4. Macklin, "Dignity is a Useless Concept," p. 1420.
5. *Ibid.*, 1419–1420.

6. Dignitas, http://news.bbc.co.uk/1/hi/world/europe/2676837.stm.

7. D. Callahan, "When Self-Determination Runs Amok," *Hastings Center Report*, 22:2 (1992), pp. 52–5.

8. *Cf.* John Harris, "In Vitro Fertilisation: The Ethical Issues (I)," *The Philosophical Quarterly*, 132 (1983), pp. 217–237.

9. R. Hertz, *Death and the Right Hand as an Anthropological Study of Different Cultural Ideas about Death* (Aberdeen: Cohen & West, 1960).

10. Martha C. Nussbaum, *Hiding from Humanity* (Princeton: Princeton University Press, 2004), p. 6.

11. Häyry, "Another Look at Dignity," p. 10.

12. US President's Council on Bioethics first report *Human Cloning and Human Dignity* (2002).

13. *Ibid.*, p. 4.

14. Søren Holm, "A Life in the Shadow: One Reason Why We Should Not Clone Humans," *Cambridge Quarterly of Healthcare Ethics*, 7:2 (1998), pp. 160–162; A. Colman, "Why Human Cloning Should Not be Attempted," *The Genetic Revolution and Human Rights*, ed. Justine Burley (Oxford: Oxford University Press, 1999), p. 15.

15. E.g. Häyry, "Another Look at Dignity"; S. Wilkinson, *Bodies for Sale: Ethics and Exploitation in the Human Body Trade* (London: Routledge, 2003).

16. Nuffield Council on Bioethics, *Genetics and Human Behaviour* (2002).

17. *Ibid.*, p. 121.

18. Häyry, "Another Look at Dignity"; D. Pullman, "Universalism, Particularism and the Ethics of Dignity," *Christian Bioethics*, 7:3 (2001), pp. 333–358.

19. Via Romana, http://www.novaroma.org/via_romana/.

20. Cicero, *De officiis,* I. 30, trans. Walter Miller, ed. Loeb (Cambridge: Harvard University Press, 1913).

21. *Hamlet* (II, ii, 115-117).

22. Thomas Hobbes, *Leviathan* (1651), ed. C. B. Macpherson (Harmondsworth: Penguin Books, 1983), pp. 151–152.

23. Primo Levi, *If This is a Man & The Truce* (London: Abacus, 1993), p. 96.

24. V. E. Frankl, *Man's Search for Meaning*, transl. I. Lasch (Hodder and Stoughton, 1974).

25. I. Illich, *Limits to Medicine: Medical Nemesis: The Expropriation of Health*, (Harmondsworth: Penguin Books, 1976).

26. T. Parsons, *The Social System*, (London: Routledge and Kegan Paul, 1951).

27. T. Szasz, *The Myth of Mental Illness*, (London: Paladin, 1964).

28. E. Goffman, *Asylums: Essays on the Social Situations of Mental Patients and Other Inmates*, (New York: Anchor Books, 1961).

29. M. Foucault, *The Birth of the Clinic*, (London: Tavistock, 1973).

30. S. Sontag, *Illness as Metaphor and Aids and its Metaphors*. (New York: Picador, 2001).

31. Häyry, "Another Look at Dignity," p. 12.

32. *E.g.*, K. D. Clouser and B. Gert, "A Critique of Principlism," *Journal of Medicine and Philosophy*, 15:2 (1999), pp. 219–36; Søren Holm, "Not Just Autonomy—The Principles of American Biomedical Ethics," *Journal of Medical Ethics*, 21 (1995), pp. 332–338.

Nine

AUTONOMY
(AND A LITTLE BIT OF DIGNITY)
IN BIOETHICS

Niall Scott

1. Introduction

Autonomy and dignity are a much debated subjects in bioethics, especially where bioethics is focused on the concerns of the treatment of human beings in biomedical ethics, rather than the broader interest of bioethics with regard to non-human animals and ecosystems. Some of Professor Häyry's work in bioethics is devoted to an understanding of the concepts of autonomy and dignity and the role they play in a utilitarian bioethics, more specifically in biomedical ethics. In this paper I will discuss some of what I take to be Häyry's ideas concerning autonomy in his writings and work done with Tuija Takala. I aim to provide a response that defends a Kantian understanding of autonomy and dignity. Häyry's approach to autonomy and dignity is quite varied. In one place Häyry rejects the idea of autonomy in favor of freedom.[1] In others he uses the concept in a utilitarian approach,[2] and elsewhere in investigating a European approach to bioethics[3] where he might have used autonomy, he opts for a discussion based on dignity, solidarity and precaution as possible crucial themes to build a bioethics around.

2. What is Autonomy?

Autonomy is to be generally understood as the capacity for self determination and the ability to act on freely chosen principles. Although its definition is traceable to Kant, in bioethics, there are several different approaches to autonomy, which form part of interesting and challenging debates on how we ought to treat people in the biomedical context.

Autonomy in utilitarian thought is functional in that it ought to be promoted as a value in so far as it maximizes happiness or delivers the required consequences of a given act. A utilitarian idea of autonomy and dignity treats them as malleable concepts through which it is possible to access the worth of a person, and as a result how, once worth has been measured how that person can be treated. So it is a route to treatment rather than a fundamental reason for treating a person in a particular manner. Furthermore, Häyry's perspective on autonomy and dignity seems to be such that the meaning of the term itself should serve utility; in other words the definition or notion can be altered to address the requirements of a utilitarian endeavor.[4] This use of autonomy explains in part his rejection of it in favor of freedom and elsewhere his acceptance of it in some situations regarding consent.[5] It is quite different from autonomy and dignity being established as a grounding for the treatment of others, as is found in the Kantian approach, which I will outline below. Even Beauchamp and Childress' well known Principalist approach to biomedical ethics treats autonomy as capturing a range of expressions that "need to be refined in light of particular objectives."[6] Thus they are wanting, like Häyry to allow the concept to be amendable with particular goals in mind, as long as the general features of liberty and agency remain. For Beauchamp and Childress, the principle of autonomy ought not to be allowed priority over the other principles of beneficence, non-maleficence and justice. It is a principle they claim focuses on autonomous choice rather than the autonomous person.[7] As a result, like in Häyry's utilitarian view the emphasis on choice leads to autonomy being discussed with regard to particular situations. Instead, Kant provides us with a general theory as to what autonomy *is* and why it ought to be respected, so that autonomy as a concept can speak to and inform particular situations.

3. Kantian Autonomy

In contrast to Häyry's position then, for a Kantian, autonomy forms part of the foundation of what is necessary for moral action to be possible at all, since it is a defining characteristic of humans as moral agents. For Kant, autonomy cannot simply submit to utility; it cannot be refined or altered with respect to achieving particular bioethical goals. It is a fundamental aspect of who we are.

Kant's conception of autonomy is quite deep and forms part of a complex of interrelated aspects of what a human being is as a moral agent. Furthermore, it is what outlines our moral obligation to others and to ourselves. It provides a starting point for how we ought to treat other human beings and how we ought to treat ourselves, and thus it would seem a rather important point to follow in the field of bioethics and specifically biomedical ethics. For Kant, to be autonomous is to be capable of freely choosing to act on the basis of universally valid moral principles. Essential to Kant's notion of autonomy is rationality. Autonomous action involves acting on principles that are rationally binding on all human beings, as exemplified in the categorical imperative, in the formula that emphasizes humanity: "Act so that you use humanity in your own person, as well as in the person of every other, always at the same time as an end, never merely as a means."[8] The expression of autonomy in the *Groundwork* as this capacity to set moral laws which can be assented to and acted upon is: "The idea of the will of every rational being as a will giving universal laws."[9]

Crucially for Kant, autonomy is an idea, which Allen Wood notes, means that we cannot ground autonomy in "what particular rational beings might arbitrarily decree."[10] As a result we can be in error about what we think is right because we cannot reduce morality and hence autonomy to what we may think or neither can we use anything from experience to shape our understanding of it. The nature of autonomy thus does not change with regard to the consequences of an action, as it might in Häyry's utilitarian use of the concept.

For Kant autonomy and dignity are very closely related. One could say that being autonomous involves dignity in action. In the groundwork, in addition to saying something about human worth, Kant holds that autonomy is the very foundation for human dignity:

> Nothing can have a worth other than which the law determines for it. But the lawgiving itself, which determines all worth, must for that reason have dignity, that is an unconditional incomparable worth; and the word respect alone provides a becoming expression for the estimate of it that a rational being must give. Autonomy is therefore the ground of the dignity of human nature and of every rational creature.[11]

To reiterate: Kantian autonomy is part of the definition of a human being. Autonomy is the active part of dignity. Autonomy is a complex concept that feathers into a full picture of the human agent. A human can act autonomously and their autonomy can be respected.

4. Forget Freedom and Give Me Autonomy!

An important indication of Häyry's approach to autonomy is captured in his point that the notion of autonomy can be used carelessly and as a result creates conceptual problems.[12] Here, in discussing genetic information and the claim of the patient's right to know vs. the right to remain in ignorance of one's own genetic knowledge, he holds that the concept can be defined in ways such that different norms can be derived from it. Thus autonomy is a malleable concept and it can be reformulated to achieve certain ends. Where autonomy is treated as reasonable self determination, it is useful for moral agents seeking actions based on the best information available. According to Häyry and Takala, in the application of informed consent as a principle, then in order to act autonomously, a patient ought to have full access to all information available in order to be able to make a decision regarding their own welfare.[13] This puts a heavy burden of disclosure on the physician, including information that would allow the patient to reject treatment. Häyry and Takala hold that a patient cannot appeal to this conception of autonomy to give them both a right to be informed and a right to not be informed.[14] Their request is based on a demand for consistency.

I hold that in a Kantian understanding of autonomy, a patient wishing to be informed in order to make a decision about a particular procedure that they may be subject to involves several things. There is a demand being made concerning the general respect for rational decision making and there is the demand to respect the individual patient's decision making regarding their particular case. Thus a patient can make a poor decision that may go against their goal of health, or seem entirely irrational. For example, a patient may refuse pain relief, despite a procedure being very painful. I may choose, in a display of bravado, to not receive an injection at the dentist, even after I am told that the procedure will cause a great deal of pain. I may reject life saving surgery in favor of knowingly choosing a painful, slow decline in health as a result of cancer. Such a decision may be based on not receiving adequate information or involve not fully understanding the procedure available. I may even make such a decision being fully informed and understanding the procedure, but am willing to undergo some suffering, regardless of the pain relief available. Despite what appears as an irrational decision ignoring the information provided, or a decision made based on inadequate information, a patient can none the less still have their autonomy respected.

But in what sense are we committed to respecting the patient's autonomy if we appeal to Kant? It may seem that we would be committed to respecting the general decision making capacity of the patient and also respect the particular decisions that the patient makes, even if these are non-autonomous decisions. We may be confronted with the difficulty that a patient believes that they are making an autonomous decision, but they are mistaken about their conception of autonomy and what it means, if Kant's concept of autonomy were to be taken as definitive. This seems to present us with a problem of inconsistency for the Kantian position in that we are respecting a general capacity for autonomy and also respecting the non-autonomous decision of the patient. The reason for seeing this as inconsistent can have to do with a relationship between autonomy and freedom. In doing so a particular approach to freedom is being invoked, that links autonomous action to non-interference with decisions. This is the very problem that Häyry and Takala try to address and they argue that one cannot pair Kantian autonomy with a Millian conception of freedom.

Häyry and Takala propose a Millian conception of autonomy which suggests that "individuals are entitled to make their own decisions on whatever grounds they wish, as long as they do not inflict harm on others by these decisions."[15] Häyry considers the two positions, that of Kant and Mill to be competing. The Millian view of autonomy as freedom given above, paired with dignity, is incompatible with the Kantian view of autonomy. Certainly this is true; these positions are not only competing, but incompatible. Combinations of them—Millian autonomy paired with Kantian dignity are bound to cause serious problems, as pointed out above. Thus a Millian conception of freedom is mixed up with a Kantian conception of autonomy when we try to both respect the capacity for autonomy (Kant) and to respect the individual's particular non-autonomous decision (granting freedom). However, respecting an individual's particular decisions in granting freedom, does not necessarily respect their autonomy.

I think it is possible to contend that Mill's conception of freedom is not properly concerned with personal autonomy at all. Mill does not use the term himself to describe his position. For Mill's conception of freedom to be effective, it needs to be balanced by a conception of dignity. The Kantian conception of general respect for autonomy does not require anything in addition. Since Kant sees autonomy and free agency to be the same thing, when an agent is acting non-autonomously, they are not acting freely. So, if I refuse pain relief when I go to the dentist, no matter whether it is informed or not informed, my decision is irrational and will result in considerable suffering to myself. On a Kantian model, perhaps we have grounds for saving the inconsistency thrown up above and interfere with the non autonomous, unfree decision being made.

5. Forget Freedom and Give Me Cannabis!

With regard to Kant it would be wrong to treat these (autonomy and dignity) as two entirely different concepts. Instead one is an expression of the other, as I have presented above. Thus, where Häyry argues that the Kantian conception of dignity cannot sit well with a Millian conception of autonomy, i.e. that we can do and be what ever we want and we ought to be given absolute moral worth he is correct. However Häyry claims that Kant tried to merge two incompatible concepts and lost much in the process.[16] What he claims Kant lost was the opportunity to provide an argument for respecting the autonomy in terms of actual empirical choices that people make. So Kant's application of the categorical imperative forbidding suicide and perhaps hence euthanasia, or the selling of organs as immoral is done at the expense of "individual self governance," or "autonomy" as it is usually understood in present day ethical discussions.[17] The very reason though that Kant sees these as immoral is that they involve a person acting heteronomously *not* autonomously. Häyry's appeal to "autonomy as it is usually understood in present day discussions" involves shifting his argument from Kant's understanding of autonomy to present day understandings of autonomy. What is actually lost instead then is all of Kant's understanding of autonomy, which I think we could do well with keeping, as it provides the very difficult challenge of why we ought to respect the idea of autonomy in a person or humanity in general irrespective of what an individual person may want for themselves at a particular time and place. As a result, the

Kantian position on autonomy leads to accepting a realist morality, such that there are simply some things that will remain immoral. For instance, not permitting an individual to sell organs is a restriction that is worth keeping, as it prevents exploitation. Organ *donation* on the other hand may well be permissible, but not required. The moral permissibility of organ donation, in addition to benefiting the recipient restoratively, also promotes autonomy in both the donor and recipient and the duty of beneficence. I admit that this is no easy discussion to engage with, and further argument is necessary with regard to autonomy.

In a complete rejection of autonomy in favor of freedom, Häyry sensationally claims that "respect for the autonomy of persons can lead to disrespect as regards their individual liberty."[18] In considering the use of cannabis as a pain killer, he argues that the Kantian approach to autonomy would demand that the use of cannabis would have to conform to the demands of the categorical imperative and that Kantians may object to its use because of the negative effect cannabis can have on rational decision making. In this example he claims to show that Kantian autonomy can restrict freedom. However, it may well be the case that the example does not concern a moral issue at all, but one of prudence, or at least a means end reasoning process that Kant would treat as a hypothetical imperative. This would be an imperative of the form if I want x I ought to do y. It would be a mistake then to think that the general respect for autonomy is offended or damaged by the prudential reasoning involved in what kind of pain killer to use. We can give practical reasons for the use of cannabis as an effective treatment for the relief of pain and avoid over moralizing such cases. The general duty to respect autonomy still stands.

What becomes apparent is that it may well be the case that in upholding autonomy, one might end up restricting an individual's freedom. We are not restricting autonomy's freedom, but licentious freedom, which is a different thing. I can see no problem with this. In the essay "An Answer to the Question: What is Enlightenment?" Kant makes this point clear, that it is permissible and even necessary to restrict freedom for certain societal and individual goals to be possible, but this does not restrict autonomy, drawing a distinction between the private and the public use of reason: "A citizen cannot refuse to pay the taxes imposed upon him; an impertinent censure of such levies when he is to pay them may even be punished as a scandal (which could occasion general insubordination). But the same citizen expresses his thoughts about the inappropriateness or injustice of such decrees."[19]

In this chapter I have defended a Kantian view of autonomy and a little bit of dignity. In this view autonomy can be respected and freedoms can be limited. Kant's conception of autonomy and Häyry's conception of autonomy appear to be about different things—the former is about the state of the human the agent and the latter about the extent to which certain freedoms ought to be permitted in order to achieve particular goals. In other words, the latter is a procedure that can be adjusted to suit the goals—such as the need for pain relief—that are desired. This is of course an important matter in a caring approach to patient welfare. It may well be that many particular situations that invoke moral arguments concerning the use of freedom are practical problems rather than moral. Whether or not a person's freedom is advanced or restricted does not need to come into conflict with the concept of autonomy as a definitional feature of the human agent.

NOTES

1. Matti Häyry, "Forget Autonomy and Give me Freedom!" *Bioethics and Social Reality*, ed. Matti Häyry, Tuija Takala and Peter Herisssone-Kelly (Amsterdam: Rodopi, 2005), pp. 31–35.

2. Matti Häyry and Tuija Takala, "Genetic Information, Rights and Autonomy," *Theoretical Medicine and Bioethics*, 22 (September 2001), pp. 403–414.

3. Matti Häyry, "European Values in Bioethics: Why, What and How to Be Used?" *Theoretical Medicine and Bioethics*, 24 (May 2003), pp. 199–214.

4. Häyry and Takala, "Genetic Information, Rights and Autonomy," p. 411.

5. Matti Häyry, "Prescribing Cannabis: Freedom, Autonomy and Values," *Journal of Medical Ethics*, 30 (2004), pp. 333–336.

6. Tom L. Beauchamp and James F. Childress, *Principles of Biomedical Ethics* 5th ed. (Oxford: Oxford University Press, 2001), p. 58.

7. *Ibid.*

8. Immanuel Kant, *Groundwork to the Metaphysics of Morals* in *Practical Philosophy*, ed. Mary J. Gregor, *Cambridge Edition of the Works of Immanuel Kant* (Cambridge: Cambridge University Press, 1996), G 4:429, p. 80.

9. *Ibid.*, G: 4:431, p. 81.

10. Allen Wood, *Kant's Ethical Thought* (Cambridge: Cambridge University Press, 1999), p. 157.

11. Immanuel Kant, *Groundwork to the Metaphysics of Morals*, G 4:436, p. 85.

12. Matti Häyry and Tuija Takala, "Genetic Information, Rights and Autonomy," p. 410.

13. *Ibid.*, p. 411.

14. *Ibid.*

15. *Ibid.*

16. Matti Häyry, "The Tension Between Self-Governance and Absolute Inner Worth in Kant's Moral Philosophy," *Journal of Medical Ethics*, 31 (2005), pp. 645–647, p. 646.

17. *Ibid.*

18. Matti Häyry, "Forget Autonomy and Give me Freedom!" p. 31.

19. Immanuel Kant, "An Answer to the Question: What is Enlightenment?" *Kant's Political Writings* (Cambridge: Cambridge University Press, 1992), 8:37, p. 19.

Ten

CONCEPTS AND DEFINITIONS OF THE PRECAUTIONARY PRINCIPLE: AN ETHICAL ANALYSIS

Michael Parker and Paolo Vineis

1. Introduction

Risk and uncertainty are important considerations in scientific research and in the making of policy about the uses of science and technology. A key question for policy-makers concerns how best to respond appropriately to risk and uncertainty when they arise as factors in decision-making. An increasingly common claim is that policy-makers ought to adopt an approach guided by what has come to be known as the "precautionary principle." In this chapter we consider some of the ethical underpinnings of this principle, and explore some of its implications. There is a voluminous and expanding literature on the precautionary principle and a corresponding proliferation of definitions.[1] A generic version might read something like the following:

> Where a course of action (e.g. a technological innovation) presents a "possible" (or, "credible," "plausible," "likely" or "foreseeable") risk of a "substantial" (or "serious") "harm" (or, "threat" or "damage"), that action (or innovation) should be avoided—even where there is no conclusive evidence that the harm (or damage) will result from the action.

The precautionary principle has been called upon in a number of different contexts. As the definition above suggests, this has often been when the introduction of a new technology or product has been proposed, for instance, gene therapy, the use of genetically modified organisms (GMOs), pesticides, or dyes and so on and where there has been concern that this may pose a danger to the environment or to human health.[2] Recent experience provides good grounds for believing such an approach might be appropriate in many contexts. It has become clear in recent years for example, that there have been many cases in which early warnings, had they been correctly interpreted (that is, with precaution in mind), would have avoided considerable harms. For example, the United States had very few cases of limb defects from Thalidomide, compared to other countries, because Frances Kelsey, an officer at the US Food and Drug Administration, delayed approval of the drug. Both Kelsey and Lenz in Germany (who came too late, since he described as many as 4,000 babies with malformations) endured a great deal of criticism in the name of the "objectivity" of medicine at the time and faced threats to their professional credibility.[3] And yet, their precautionary actions, in particular those of Kelsey, can be seen in retrospect to have avoided significant harms. It is plausible given evidence of this kind to claim that the general adoption of the precautionary principle in technology assessment would result in a significant reduction in harms and be a reasonable basis upon which to build policy. In this chapter we explore this claim.

2. Definitions and Principles

In considering the coherence of the precautionary principle and its suitability as a guiding principle in public policy two sets of questions are of relevance. The first of these concerns the definition of key terms within the principle. How for example, ought one to define terms such as "harm," "damage," and "threat"? What does it mean for a harm to be "serious" or "significant" and is there a difference between the two? What is a "high," "plausible" or "credible" risk of such harm occurring? And, finally, what is to constitute "certainty," "conclusive evidence," "justification" or "good reason"? Key to addressing this particular set of concerns will be consideration of related questions about who ought to be involved in the processes of reaching agreement about what is to count, for example, as a "serious harm," that is, the making of value judgments in this area, and what kinds of social and political processes would be appropriate to the making of such decisions? Despite its importance, the definitions of key terms informing the precautionary principle will not be the main focus of this chapter. We shall however return to some related issues i.e. those concerning the role of public reason and deliberation in the making of policy at one or two places and in our conclusions.[4]

In this chapter we focus instead on a second set of questions about the precautionary principle. These concern the *coherence* and the *scope* of the moral principles and claims upon which the principle rests. We argue that in addition to raising difficult questions about the definition of key terms such as "risk" (including the question of how decisions about what is acceptable should be made) the precautionary principle draws heavily upon two moral claims: that there is an overriding duty to avoid harms, and that there is a moral distinction between acts and omissions. The first of these is a form of "negative utilitarianism," which requires that in policy decisions about technological innovation the primary concern ought to be the *avoidance of harm* rather than, say, the promotion of *benefits*: reference to benefits being noticeable by its absence from the definition of the principle with which we began this chapter. The second of these claims is that there is an intrinsic moral distinction between an "act" and an "omission," for instance between introducing and not introducing a technology. One way of capturing this second claim might be to say that in a situation in which the implementation of a new technology was being considered and both its implementation and its non-implementation posed indeterminate but comparable risks of harm, the precautionary principle would suggest that it would be right (precautionary) to decide *against* implementation. The justification for this is that the fact that one is an action and the other an omission marks a morally significant distinction between the two ways forward, even if the foreseeable harms are comparable. We consider each of these claims in turn and argue that whilst it may well be possible to develop a coherent account of the precautionary principle, doing so will require significant modification of the principle.

3. The Dangers of Inaction

The precautionary principle is most often called upon in situations in which the introduction of a new technology is being proposed and where this is associated with uncertainty about risks and harms. In such cases the principle is usually taken to require that a technology should *not* be introduced where it poses a significant threat, even if it cannot be conclusively shown that the threat will materialize. At first glance, this seems an eminently sensible and appropriately conservative approach to technology assessment. However, whilst the origin of the use of the principle in the setting of environmental concerns explains the tendency to emphasize restraint in the use of technology, consideration of the role of technology in other settings such as medicine e.g. in the treatment or prevention of disease, makes it clear that *failing to act* can also in many cases present a serious, even if uncertain, threat e.g. through the failure to implement important public health measures. Such cases make it clear that deciding not to act can in some cases, perhaps many, pose risks of a similar kind and magnitude to those presented by action and suggests that if policy-makers are serious about the avoidance of harms they should consider with equal seriousness the consequences both of *action and inaction*,[5] that is that the principle of precaution should be applied to all potential threats, not only to some of them. This suggests the need for a revision of the definition of the precautionary principle above to something like the following:

> Where there is a credible risk of serious harm, the action or the omission that best minimizes the likelihood of harm should be undertaken. This could, for example be achieved through the *introduction* of a public health measure or through the decision *not to introduce* a new agent—even where there is no conclusive evidence that the harm (or damage) will result from the action.

This rewording differs significantly from the ways in which the precautionary principle is currently understood. Current usage places great emphasis on the risks, uncertainties and harms associated with the introduction of new technologies, but little emphasis, if any at all, on the harms of *failing* to introduce such technologies. This is understandable given the origins of the principle in concerns about environmental damage and about cases of ill-considered innovation, but the fact remains that the avoidance of harms must surely require policy-makers to take seriously the full range of potential threats wherever they originate.

Many advocates of the precautionary principle would want to resist this conclusion however, and this revised definition, arguing that placing greater emphasis on the potential harms arising from actions rather than on those arising from omissions is justified. What grounds might there be for this claim? There are several candidates. One might for example hold the belief that the *status quo* is simply by its nature of intrinsic moral value. This is something like a claim that it is wrong to interfere with Nature. But this would be a very strange belief to hold for a number of reasons. Firstly, change in nature is inevitable and all-pervading making the idea of *status quo* in nature untenable. Furthermore, a belief in the intrinsic value and sanctity of the Natural is incompatible with the practice of medicine and of technological innovation of any kind. A second possible justification for placing greater weight on action than inaction might be one grounded in ecological arguments about the dangers of rapid ecological change (that is, that such change causes "genomic stress").[6] This is an important argument, but this justification too has its limits. Firstly, this is only an argument against *rapid* change, not against change *per se* and secondly, it is clear here too that in many cases inaction i.e. the failure to implement a technology can also lead to rapid environmental change and genetic stress. If, for example, the Thames Barrier were not to be raised during a flood warning, this would change the environment in the Thames Valley and Central London both dramatically and rapidly. And, this suggests that the absence of technological intervention may bring with it certain environmental risks and suggests too that the key concern in such situations ought to be the avoidance of harm (that is, genomic stress) and not the question of whether such harms are to be avoided by an action or inaction. Neither arguments from the sanctity of Nature, nor those about environmental shock are intrinsically arguments against the claim that the foreseeable harmful effects of both innovation and non-innovation should be taken into equal consideration in policy-making.

A third possible justification for rejecting the moral equivalence of acts and omissions might be to argue that whilst it may be true that both actions and omissions can lead to harms, there is an *intrinsic* moral distinction between them which justifies placing greater moral weight on actions than inactions irrespective of the likely consequences of so doing. Such a claim has a long history in deontological moral philosophy and in the context of the current discussion might come down to a claim that in situations in which the foreseeable harms of two courses of action are comparable in their magnitude and seriousness, it is nevertheless morally better to resist acts such as technological innovation because the causing of comparable harms through an action is intrinsically worse morally than allowing them to occur through an omission. This is a problematic position for anyone committed to the precautionary principle to hold for two reasons, both reasons arising out of the question of how much weight, in decision-making, is to be put on the moral status of the distinction. If some, any, weight is to be placed on the distinction it must hypothetically at least be possible for there to arise a situation in which it would be right to proceed in a way which involved a more harmful inaction than to proceed with a less harmful action. That is it must be possible for it to require one to choose the most harmful of two routes. If this is the case, the acts-omissions distinction requires the rejection of the precautionary principle at least insofar as its object is the avoidance of harms. If by contrast, no weight at all is to be placed on the acts-omissions distinction then it is irrelevant to policy-making, precautionary or otherwise, and the key policy question remains the avoidance of harms whether through action or inaction.

One response to this would be for the advocates of the precautionary principle to argue that even if no *intrinsic* moral weight should be given to the acts-omissions distinction, there is good contingent reason to be more cautious about interventions than non-interventions. Surely, it might be argued, the burden of proof ought to lie with those who wish to introduce new technologies to show that they are harmless rather than on those who wish to resist (usually the public) to prove that they are harmful. By placing the burden of proof here, the precautionary principle might be said to rightly emphasize the asymmetry between the burden of proof about safety of a technology (to be provided for instance by an industry) on the one hand and the burden of proof concerning its harmfulness (usually provided by the victims) on the other, particularly when one considers the numerous episodes in the past in which accurate testing of product safety was not performed, and it was up to the victims to provide evidence of damage in retrospect. This response has two weaknesses. The first of these is that where the burden of proof is said to rest with those who wish to show that there is no harm, this ought surely to apply equally to those who wish to introduce a technology and those who do not. This implies that those who argue that not introducing a technology is harmless must also be required to show why they believe this to be the case. If on the other hand the burden of proof rests with those who wish to show harm, this too ought surely to be required of both intervening and not intervening. A second weakness of requiring those who claim harmlessness to bear the burden of proof is that it is notoriously difficult to prove a negative i.e. to show that a certain exposure is harmless. This derives from the fact that (a) very large numbers of observations are needed to exclude a small excess of a rare outcome, and (b) some outcomes (for example cancer) have a very long latency period before becoming manifest.

Despite these weaknesses however, there are at least two reasons why in our view it will often be right to place greater emphasis on understanding and taking into account the potential harms of innovation. The first of these is because in a great many cases, but not all, those who wish to innovate are going to be much more powerful and richer than those who wish to resist it, having more resources available to develop and make their case. This does not mean that technological innovation should always be rejected, but it does mean that it is vital that any decision-making process has adequate built in protections. One of these protections might be a requirement for those who wish to innovate to provide a very high standard of evidence and for such evidence to be independently assessed. Another protection might be the use of public resources to investigate potential harms whether caused by act or omission The second reason why it might be reasonable to place more emphasis on the potential harms of innovation is that in many cases the evidence provided by experience will mean that the likely effects of inaction can be known with a greater degree of certainty than those of the proposed innovation.

4. The Importance of Benefits

But should policy-makers be negative utilitarians at all? Should the default position in technology assessment be the avoidance of harms? It is striking to note that the definition of the precautionary principle with which we began this chapter included no explicit reference to the potential benefits of technological innovation or of a requirement to balance the potential harms of such technology against potential benefits. Intuitively, this seems an unbalanced approach to policy-making. There seems no good reason why the consideration of the implications of introducing a technology should only take account of its potential harms and not of its potential benefits, particularly when in most cases those who argue in favor of a technological innovation do so explicitly on the basis of claims about its benefits. Whilst policy-makers ought of course always to retain a healthy degree of skepticism with regard to claims about potential benefits, particularly when these claims are made by those with commercial or political interests at stake, it is nevertheless true in at least some cases that the introduction of a technology does indeed offer benefits. Where this is the case, they are surely of ethical significance and of relevance to policy.

Just as skepticism of the kind suggested above, is important, an assessment of the balance between risks and benefits of a technology must also be capable of taking into account the fact that one can often easily perceive and be seduced by the benefits of technology, overlooking potential harms. Such harms are often only picked up much later and even then with difficulty. For example, several drugs have been introduced because they had obvious benefits, only for late-developing and rare side-effects to become apparent many years after introduction (like with cerivostatin, Vioxx). The benefits tend to increase as the frequency of the outcomes that are meant to be prevented increases, whereas harms are independent of such frequency. This principle is illustrated in Figure 1. For example, prescribing statins to patients with very high levels of cholesterol is associated with a much lower Number Needed to Treat than treating patients with lower levels, but the side-effects arise independently of cholesterol levels. Therefore, a threshold can be identified below which treatment is not advised.

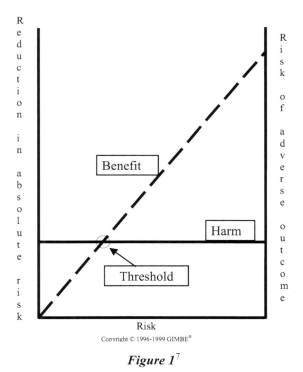

Figure 1[7]

Notwithstanding the need for skepticism about benefits and caution about the dangers of overestimating the benefits of innovation, policy-makers, confronted by technologies with a perceived uncertainty and risk ought to consider evidence, where this is available, both about their potential harms and benefits and come to a judgment on a case by case basis about whether the potential risks are worth taking in order to secure the potential benefits. This suggests the need for a further redrafting of our precautionary principle along something like the following lines.

> Where there is a perceived serious threat, an action or an omission should be chosen in the light of a consideration of both of the potential harms *and benefits* associated with each. Such a decision, to be precautionary, should pay particular attention to the achievement of an appropriate "balance" between harms and benefits—even where there is no conclusive evidence that the harm (or damage) will result from the action.

In practice of course the precautionary principle, even as defined at the start of this chapter, does take *some* implicit account of benefits in that it is only, even by its advocates, considered to apply where the potential harms are thought to be significant, serious or substantial i.e. not to all interventions. And this implies that interventions in the pursuit of benefits are implicitly acceptable insofar as their foreseeable or perceived harms are not serious, significant or, substantial. So, even if the pursuit of benefits is not explicitly required by the precautionary principle, it does at least imply that the pursuit of benefits through technological innovation ought to be tolerated where its perceived side-effects pose only minimal risks of harm.

The considerations above suggest however, that this minimal position is incoherent and that the assessment of the ethical implications of technological innovation ought to take into account evidence about the full range of potential benefits and harms. Whatever decision-making process is adopted, one consideration any such process will need to address is the question of whether there are ever situations in which the risk of a serious harm might be legitimately taken in the pursuit of important benefits? It seems likely that the answer to this question must be yes even if such occasions will be rare. A good analogy might be the acceptance in medicine that it is on occasion right to subject patients to the possibility of potentially serious harms e.g. death, in the pursuit of cures e.g. through surgery or chemotherapy. Similar choices need to be made at the level of policy for example in public health where the public benefits of, say vaccination programmes, need to be weighed up against the knowledge that in some cases particular individuals will come to very serious harm through this intervention.

And this implies that policy-making in relation to new technology will not always be precautionary, except insofar as this is taken to mean that there is a requirement to reach moral judgments on the basis of well-informed and relatively cautious consideration of the foreseeable harms and benefits. This means that it will not always be wrong to knowingly choose to take a risk of a serious harm in the pursuit of benefits. It will however, be of vital importance in all cases for those who make such decisions to do so in the light of a healthy skepticism about claims about benefits and an awareness of the role of power and of vested interests in such claims.

5. Conclusion

We began this chapter by emphasizing the unavoidability of considerations of risk and uncertainty in policy-making about the uses of science and technology. It has been suggested that an appropriate response to such uncertainty would be to adopt what has come to be known as a "precautionary" approach. We have argued that current versions of the precautionary principle rest upon two contestable claims: that policy should be oriented towards the avoidance of harms rather than towards the achievement of benefits; and that a moral distinction ought to be made between acts and omissions. We have discussed these two claims and have argued that both are questionable. We have also argued that the making of policy concerning the use of science and technology needs to consider both potential benefits and harms of innovations and this will involve the making of a moral judgment. We have also argued that such judgments ought to be neutral about acts and omissions, that is, between the introduction and non-introduction of technology. Whilst it is essential that policy-makers retain a skeptical attitude towards claims about benefits (and harms), because both harms and benefits are uncertain and claims are often made by those with a vested interest, this does not mean that such claims are of no moral significance. This does not imply a rejection of precaution in science policy. Indeed, it implies that a precautionary approach to science and technology is both appropriate and required. Our argument suggests however that a truly precautionary model will require all morally relevant considerations to be taken account of in decision-making.

We have also suggested that, in addition to problems concerning the *coherence* of the moral principles underlying the precautionary approach, the making of precautionary policy in science and technology will also need to pay attention to consideration of the definition of the key terms i.e. what is to count as a harm? What does it mean for a harm or threat to be "significant" or "serious"? What is to qualify as "certainty" or "reasonable evidence"? And, importantly too, the central importance of reaching political agreement about these essentially contested concepts raises the political question of who should be involved in deciding what is to count as "acceptable risk," "serious harm," and so on? And this in turn raises the question of what model of decision-making should underpin the precautionary approach? What role is to be given to "experts," to politicians, to the people who will be affected by decisions, to the population at large, and so on? These are ultimately political questions. We believe that a truly precautionary approach to science and technology requires policy to be made through genuinely participatory and deliberative processes of public reason.

NOTES

1. C. Cranor, "Toward Understanding Aspects of the Precautionary Principle," *Journal of Medicine and Philosophy*, 27: 3 (2002), pp. 259–279; H. T. Engelhardt and F. Jotterand, "The Precautionary Principle: A Dialectical Reconsideration," *Journal of Medicine and Philosophy*, 27:3 (2002), pp. 301–312; John Harris and Søren Holm, "Extending Human Lifespan and the Precautionary Paradox," *Journal of Medicine and Philosophy*, 27:3 (2002), pp. 355–368; D. Resnik, "The Precautionary Principle and Medical Decision Making," *Journal of Medicine and Philosophy*, 27:3 (2002), pp. 281–299; D. Weed, "Precaution, Prevention and Public Health Ethics," *Journal of Medicine and Philosophy*, 27:3 (2002), pp. 313–332; Matti Häyry, "Precaution and Solidarity," *Cambridge Quarterly of Healthcare Ethics*, 14 (2005): 199–206.

2. D. Kriebel, J. Tickner, P. Epstein, J. Lemons, R. Levins, E. L. Loechler, M. Quinn, R. Rudel, T. Schettler and M. Stoto, "The Precautionary Principle in Environmental Science," *Environmental Health Perspectives*, 109:9 (2001), pp. 871–876.

3. A. Daemmrich, "A Tale of Two Experts: Thalidomide and Political Engagement in the United States and West Germany," *Social History of Medicine*, 15:1 (2002), pp. 137–157.

4. D. Kriebel and J. Tickner, "Reenergizing Public Health through Precaution," *American Journal of Public Health*, 91:9 (September 2001), pp. 1351–1355.

5. Engelhardt and Jotterand, "The Precautionary Principle: A Dialectical Reconsideration," pp. 301–312; Harris and Holm, "Extending Human Lifespan and the Precautionary Paradox," pp. 355–368; Matti Häyry, "Precaution and Solidarity."

6. Paolo Vineis, "Scientific Basis for the Precautionary Principle," *Toxicology and Applied Pharmacology*, 207:2, suppl. 1 (2005), pp. 658–662.

7. P. P. Glasziou and L. M. Irwig, "An Evidence-Based Approach to Individualising Treatment," *British Medical Journal*, 311:7016 (18 November 1995), pp. 1356–1359.

Eleven

JUSTICE OR SOLIDARITY? THINKING ABOUT NORDIC PRIORITIZATION IN THE LIGHT OF RAWLS

Vilhjálmur Árnason

1. Introduction

In his article "European Values in Bioethics: Why, What and How to Be Used?" Matti Häyry asks whether the "principles of *dignity*, *precaution* and *solidarity* reflect the European ethos better than the liberal concepts of autonomy, harm and justice."[1] He voices sensible doubts about that and shows how open to different interpretations these principles are. In this chapter, I will attempt to show how the main principles of recent reports on prioritization in the Nordic health care systems exemplify this complexity. I argue that although the principle of solidarity is a key notion of these reports, they involve a mode of thought that seems to be in line with a Rawlsian conception of justice.

This is not surprising since the Nordic systems aim at securing health care as a primary good for everyone, and protecting in particular the interests of the worst off, while Rawls's contract theory reconciles the individual motivation to protect one's interests with the requirement to secure social reciprocity protected by institutions.

2. The Principle of Welfare—Genesis and Validity

The underlying principle of socialized systems of health care in the Nordic countries could be labeled as an egalitarian welfare principle. It is instructive in this regard to look at the first article of the Icelandic law on health care:

> Every citizen is to have access to the most perfect health-care services that at each time is possible to provide in order to protect mental, physical and social health. (Act no. 59/1983)

The intention of this law is to provide everyone with equal right to health care. This is a positive welfare right which creates duties on behalf of the state to provide each citizen, indiscriminately, with the best health care available at each point in time.

Historically, this was extremely important in order to improve and equalize the life conditions of people. Only a few decades ago, the public suffered
from grave injustice, partly because individuals were not secured the basic
rights that we now take for granted in our welfare system. The national health
care act was a major stepping stone towards securing that everyone in Icelandic society would be provided with the basic goods necessary for each citizen to project his or her own plan of life. There was a broad political agreement about this policy which guaranteed the citizens a much fairer equality of
opportunity than before. At the same time it substantiated solidarity in the
sense that the citizens are jointly responsible for one another and will not tolerate that someone will miss the opportunities in life because of bad luck in
the natural lottery of health or because of accidents.

From this historical perspective, the egalitarian principle of right to welfare has clearly been most valuable. It is questionable, however, whether it is a
fruitful guideline for the recent task of setting limits to health care. We must
also ask whether it has really brought about optimal health services. In order to
answer this question it must be evaluated according to what I call the three
criteria of good health care:

  – the economic criterion of (cost-)*efficiency*
  – the professional criterion of *quality*
  – the ethical criterion of *justice*

I will argue that a health care system based on the egalitarian principle of right
to welfare has to some extent failed on all accounts.

First, it is not cost-efficient. Most states are now setting limits to the sky-
rising costs of health care. This is not least because in a scheme of equal rights
of all to the best health care, there are no rational limits. This could work in a
situation of affluence, but it is insufficient in a situation of scarcity. (I leave
out the question here how much a nation can spend on health care. The only
rule that might apply here is that a nation is not to spend so much on health
care that it is unable to uphold other institutions, such as of education, necessary to provide for equal opportunities of the citizens.) We are used to think
that progress eliminates scarcity. But in the context of health care, it is a well
known fact that scarcity increases along with social progress because it is relative to historical possibilities each time. The problem is that the "cost of human ingenuity applied to health care exceeds the capacity to pay for it."[2]

Secondly, our health care system does not guarantee optimal quality of
health care. Major emphasis has been on the expansion of technologized hospital care at the neglect of prevention, self-help and traditional forms of care.
Therefore, it has not contributed well enough to the major goals of health care,
which is the protection of health and the prevention of sickness. This is a
complicated issue which has various explanations. Partly the situation is created by the "ideology" and the vision especially of the medical profession to-

wards its subject matter. Medical doctors have become increasingly special-ized in the various parts of the human body which has enabled them to get an ever increasing mastery over sickness, but this has diverted their attention from the causes of sickness and the context of disease, therapy and recovery. This is one reason why the shaping of health policy is not to be left only up to the health professionals who are likely to confuse their individual and narrow professional interests with the public interest. However, this policy appears to be supported by the public who mostly prefer to lead unhealthy lives and then be saved in hospitals when the need arises. At the same time, health is made an absolute value by these same individuals who "make ever increasing demands on the qualities and possibilities of the health cares system."[3] Consequently, the health care system seems to increase in a relatively autonomic way, driven more by the technological imperative of doing whatever is possible than by a sensible standard of good health care.

Thirdly, our health care system has not contributed well enough to a fair equality of opportunity among the citizens. To mention one reason: The fact that we get an equal chance of being cured once ill does not compensate us for our unequal chances of becoming ill.[4] Moreover, the vision of technologized medicine threatens to discriminate among patients, giving priority to those with health care problems that lend themselves to technological solutions. In this way and others, there is always an implicit hidden rationing and prioritiz-ing of health care—one that is not explicitly put forth and thrown into an open public discussion. This is a major reason why explicit prioritization should be attempted. A successful prioritization is a matter of justice, because it requires that policy decisions are made according to publicly available criteria which can be openly debated and assessed. Otherwise, the prioritization is more likely to be arbitrary, concealed and subject to private interests. A successful prioritization is a way to secure that everyone can have a necessary health care service when the need arises, that money is effectively used and that profes-sional criteria are employed in order to define and demarcate the health care services that should be financed by the state.

3. Nordic Plans of Prioritization

In recent years, Nordic nations have systematically undertaken the task to form publicly available criteria of a fair prioritization in health care. Although the conclusions are of various types, it is nevertheless possible to discern some common key features.[5] I will now try to briefly summarize the most conspicu-ous ethical standards or principles in the Nordic reports, without trying to ex-haust the principles used or making any attempt to critically assess them.

A. Human Dignity or Equal Respect

It is not surprising that this principle is the foundation of reasoning about just health care. The idea of moral equality of the citizens is literally undisputed in moral and political philosophy of our time, although there are disagreements about how best to observe it.[6] It implies the minimal requirement that health care must not discriminate between people on a-medical grounds, i.e. that patients shall receive similar treatment for comparable illnesses, independent of social status, age, income or other accidental factors. This principle also implies that people shall have equal access to health care services, regardless of where they happen to live in the country. In the Danish report, equal access is related to "formal equality approach" while "a solidarity approach may require us to compensate those who are underprivileged."[7]

B. Solidarity

The principle of equal respect as it is understood in the Nordic prioritization reports already seems to harbor a notion of solidarity. According to the Swedish report, solidarity "means not only equal opportunities of care but also an effort to equalize the outcome of care as far as possible. ... Solidarity also means devoting special considerations to the needs of the weakest, e.g. those who are not aware of their human dignity, those who have less chance than others of making their voices heard or exercising their rights."[8] In the Danish report, it is stated about solidarity that "help should be given to those that need it, and the greater and more acute the need the greater is society's, that is, all of our obligation to give it."[9] This implies that individuals are not only responsible for themselves but also co-responsible for their fellow citizens, and especially for the underprivileged. In practice, this makes itself manifest in the fact that health care is publicly financed but not merely by those individuals who use the services each time. This is well put in a Dutch report on prioritization: "Risk solidarity is when the healthy pay for the ill and good risks pay for the bad risks. Income solidarity is when the financially able pay for the less wealthy."[10] Thus everyone lives in the security that they can seek medical aid when they need it regardless of their ability to pay. It could be said that the dictum "From each according to ability, to each according to need,"[11] is the backbone of this idea of solidarity. Special emphasis is placed on securing the health care of those groups of people who have a weak standing due to age or handicap.

C. Medical Need

This principle is implied in the principle of solidarity as it is understood in the Nordic prioritization reports. This is most obvious in the Swedish report which conflates them into "The Principle of Need and Solidarity."[12] Health care needs are of various sorts and it is a matter of justice and solidarity that those who have the gravest health care need should have priority. Eric Matthews distinguishes desires and needs and argues that people have a legitimate claim only to have their needs met.[13] The problem is, however, to determine which are "the gravest health care needs" and to find out what is comparable in that regard. Most recommendations about prioritization in health care imply ideas about which services are to be emphasized above others. In the Icelandic report it says, for example:

> Priority shall be based on need for health care. The following services and forms of treatment shall have priority.
> I. Treatment of acute or life-threatening illnesses, physical or mental, and injuries which can lead to serious disability or death.
> II. Preventive health care, which has proved effective.
> The treatment of serious long-term illnesses.
> Rehabilitation and habilitation.
> Palliative terminal care.
> III. Treatment of less serious injuries, and acute and long-term illnesses of a less serious nature.
> IV. Other forms of treatment which professional experience has shown to be effective.[14]

D. Cost-Effectiveness.

This well known principle urges health care professionals to choose the less expensive option of any two that have the same effectiveness. The notion of effectiveness refers here to the benefit that an individual can receive from a particular treatment. When many people need the same treatment, it can also be a matter of justice to choose the less expensive option, even though the benefits are somewhat less for each individual, because in that way total effectiveness can be increased.[15] Futile treatment should not be provided, nor expensive treatment which has a high sacrifice cost.

E. Individual Responsibility.

In contemporary society, illnesses are increasingly related to life-style for which individuals can be said to be, at least partly, responsible. This appeal to responsibility does not mean that individuals will be charged for health care services, but rather that preventive medicine and health promotion is to be planned in the light of this fact. Moreover, some problems are such that individuals can better deal with them than the health care system. Appropriately applied, this principle harbors important potentials for constructive changes in medical practice (somewhat in line with the idea of empowerment) but these are not fleshed out in the reports and are not even mentioned in all of them.

4. Rawlsian Justice and Nordic Solidarity

Together these interrelated five standards of prioritization in the Nordic countries can be said to comprise an idea of just health care. It has been argued that the (European) principle of solidarity is quite different from the (American) liberal principle of justice. The liberal approach is said to limit itself to procedural norms of justice while solidarity assumes "the existence of publicly shared values and practices that direct collective choices."[16] Hence, Pasini and Reichlin write, this "European" approach would not

> ground solidarity, or the concern for the worst off, on the perceived self-interest of individuals acting as rational egoists, as it is the case with the liberal-neutral picture of society [the authors refer here to Rawls 1972 and Daniels 1985]; rather, rejecting the abstraction of the "liberal self," who conceives of his identity as established independently of any social relationship, it would ground solidarity on a genuine concern for the common good that stems from the recognition of the inherent relatedness of human beings within a democratic community.[17]

I have my doubts about this interesting argument. It seems to me that Rawls's theory of justice is quite compatible with the Nordic notion of solidarity and that it can even be used to improve our way of thinking about just health care. The theory reconciles well the individual motivation to protect one's interests with the requirement to secure social reciprocity protected by institutions. This is built into the key notion of Rawls's theory, the "veil of ignorance" which basically means that the contractors don't know what their social position or general condition is when they reflect upon the main principles of a just society. The veil of ignorance makes it impossible to promote one's own interests without promoting that of others. In this way it represents the moral point of view where anyone's interest is equally taken into account. As Rawls writes: "The veil of ignorance insures that no one is advantaged or disadvantaged in the choice of principles by the outcome of natural chance or the contingency of social circumstances."[18]

Rawls is often criticized for being unrealistic in his description of the veil of ignorance but, as Will Kymlicka has emphasized, "the veil of ignorance is not an expression of a theory of identity [of the unencumbered liberal self]. It is an intuitive test of fairness."[19] Moreover, the principles of justice do not require that differences in circumstances between people are uprooted or that all life opportunities are equalized. What matters is that difference in this regard be justified by showing that it is to the advantage of the worst off. This would imply, for example, that privatization of health services would only be justifiable if such a change would be to everyone's advantage in the sphere of health care. On this line of reasoning, it would not count as unfair if the rich would, as a result of privatization, be able to get a quicker access to certain services if the quality of public health care was improved as well. This aspect of Rawls's thought may not square well with the peculiarity of the Scandinavian health care where "the rich as well as the poor have traditionally made use of the publicly funded services."[20] In light of the current development, the question then boils down to whether "everyone should be equally deprived of the most expensive services"[21] in the manner of strict welfare egalitarianism or whether it is possible to improve public health care by partial privatization.

For this task I believe that Rawls's theory gives an important guidance. His counter-factual agreement which is not intended to describe anything that has taken place, lends itself remarkably well to the discussion of just health care. This is because the veil of ignorance is perfectly realistic in this sphere of life. No one can know what her/his health care needs will be next year, next month or even tomorrow for that matter. Will we be paralyzed after a car accident, bed-ridden because of cancer, or demented old people when the inevitable veil of time is lifted? And if we are overly optimistic or biased in our own case, we can apply this to our children and parents: how will they fare in the health lottery? This imaginary situation seems to lend itself well, therefore, to constructing a contractual system of solidarity which squares with the reading of Pasini and Reichlin quoted above where the interests of the worst off are protected by rational egoists.

We must not read Rawls's theory too narrowly as a contract theory and regard the principle of justice as fair simply because they are chosen under a veil of ignorance. We could also put it the other way around and say that the principles of justice are chosen under a veil of ignorance because they *are* fair. Rawls writes: "The basic intuition which underlies all my ideas and they are systematically built around, is about society as a fair system of co-operation of free equals. Justice as fairness is rooted in this idea as one of the basic components of democratic culture."[22] This rootedness of justice as fairness in democratic culture shows that even the liberal contractual system of solidarity is "founded upon a pre-contractual consensus on fundamental values."[23] In Hegelian terms we could say that the *Moralität* of contractors under a veil of ignorance is a normative test of values already shaped in the historically formed *Sittlichkeit* of the society. On this reading one can see the hypothetical contractors under a veil of ignorance choose to design a solidaristic system of health care not simply because they are rational egoists but also because they realize the dependence of individuals upon a system of social relationships and values. Rawls could, therefore, in his own way, accept Habermas's idea that justice and solidarity are two sides of the same coin: "Morality cannot protect the one without the other. It cannot protect the rights of the individual without also protecting the well-being of the community to which he belongs."[24] We should be mindful of the fact that the function of the veil of ignorance is not only to make the contractors ignorant of their own position but also to make them more knowledgeable about the human condition in general and about various individual situations. As a theoretical exercise it inspires us to imagine ourselves in the situation of the worst off and thus it motivates our vision of interdependence and reciprocity in human relations.[25] In this vein of thought, Rawlsian justice can thus also contribute to "reflexive solidarity" as described by Houtepen and ter Meulen which "implies continuous reappraisal of the way that institutions and services affect the people involved in caring practices."[26]

Norman Daniels, who has applied Rawls's theory of justice to health care,[27] fruitfully regards health as the normal functioning of the body, seen as a psycho-somatic whole, and health care needs are those necessary to achieve or maintain "species-typical normal functioning" at each point in life.[28] Impairment of this functioning reduces the range of opportunity open to the individual in the course of her life. This is most often due to causes that the individual has no control over. To the most part it is determined by a natural and social lottery. This is why health care is primarily a matter of justice; its role is to protect an individual's share of life's opportunities. Although this conclusion is a result of a quite liberal mode of thought it seems to imply a notion of solidarity that can be compared with those of the Nordic reports on prioritization discussed above.

Daniels clearly places emphasis on the *joint* responsibility of the citizens, but what about *individual* responsibility? Isn't it to be expected that a liberal notion of justice emphasizes that at the cost of solidarity? Not necessarily. Prudential contractors must seek just ways to deal with this. And since they know general facts of life, they will know how difficult it is to determine what exactly is due to voluntary decisions and what is the result of natural and social conditions. Therefore, they will not take the risk of adding injustice to injury, that is, blaming the victim by discriminating between patients once the damage is done. They will rather look for indirect ways, especially through redistribution of profit from unhealthy consumption and risk activities, like smoking and mountain climbing. Besides, they will probably want to provide themselves with some elbowroom to live dangerously, without having to pay specifically for it when they find themselves in need. However, if and when health care needs can without doubt be shown to be voluntarily caused, it is a matter of justice that special health fees be placed on such behavior in order to distribute the burden of health care costs fairly.[29]

What kind of health policy would hypothetical contractors design under a veil of ignorance? Rawls has not tried to address this question but Norman Daniels has written extensively about this issue.[30] I cannot go into Daniels' theory here, but I will briefly summarize his ideas and mention their relation to the Nordic principles of prioritization outlined above. According to Daniels it is likely that if we were to construct a system of health care under a veil of ignorance we would agree that:

> – Everyone should have equal access to services needed to maintain, restore and replace a person's normal functioning and to protect the fair share of opportunities in the course of his/her life. [Equal Respect.]
> – They would prefer a scheme which would enhance people's chance of reaching a normal life span to a scheme which reduced the chance of reaching a normal life span, but giving those reaching a normal life span an increased chance of living longer. [Solidarity.]
> – They would put emphasis on providing health care services which maintain an active meaningful life but not merely on prolonging it. [(Strong!) Solidarity.]
> – They would want the system to protect an individual's share of the normal opportunity range by reducing the risks of disease and disability, by seeking an equitable distribution of the risk of disease (e.g. by work safety regulations), and by curing disease when it arises, in this order. [Solidarity.]
> – In general they will find it more important to prevent, cure or compensate for those disease conditions which involve a greater curtailment of an individual's share of the normal opportunity range than to treat those conditions that affect it less. (This can be seen as a version of the Rawlsian principle of justice that the worst off are to have priority.) [Medical Need and Solidarity.]
> – It is not a social obligation to provide health services which arise from individual preferences and are not necessary to restore a person's normal functioning. [Individual Responsibility.]

These aspects of a hypothetical contract about health care system do not imply any specific suggestions for prioritizing health care services. But they are indicative of the mode of thought that needs to be strengthened in our task to reconstruct the health care system. This means for example that we give up the one-sided emphasis on health care on demand, backed by individual rights, and try to reach a consensus on quality care which is both just and cost-effective. The main concern of justice is to provide equality of opportunity. In the context of health care this means removing the hindrances that limit people's opportunity range and result from injury, sickness or disability, or increases their chance of suffering from these conditions. And the "worst off" in this context are those in the gravest medical need or at the greatest risk to suffer from conditions that threaten to radically reduce their share of the normal opportunity range. This places strong emphasis on the *joint* responsibility or solidarity of the citizens and in some ways even stronger than has been emphasized in Nordic systems of health care.

5. Consensus?

In dealing with macro-allocation of health care goods and the making of general health policy, it is necessary to form a social agreement about general principles. In this paper I teased out such principles from official reports about prioritization in health care from the Nordic countries. I presume that even though they are not substantiated in health care policy, such reports harbor important indicators of the citizens' views about what must guide us in this task. They could be crucial now when there is an increased admittance of the fact that unlimited application of the welfare principle can overthrow the health care system. In such situations, our alleged adherence to justice and solidarity is put to the test because we can no longer escape the task of finding out which inequalities are justifiable and which are not. I argued that in order to shape a mode of thought about the health care system which can fairly limit our access to health care goods without violating solidarity, we can look in the direction of Rawls's theory of justice as fairness. Surely, this is a *procedural* notion of justice, specifying the conditions necessary for a fair distribution of goods in society. But it can also be seen as a *critical* idea, providing a perspective from where every real agreement or consensus in society can be normatively assessed.

Moreover, such a consensus requires broad public discussion which ensures that people take responsibility for the policy made, and identify with it. Therefore, ideas put forth in official reports need to be tested in public deliberation. For this discursive task Rawls's theory may not provide sufficient guidance because it precludes the ongoing democratic dialogue where the principles of justice themselves must be open for revision.[31] Ideas of deliberative democracy and discourse ethics could be more constructive for that purpose. Nevertheless, we can learn from Rawls that in fleshing out the idea of a social consensus on health care we are bound to move from individual rights-based attitude to just general rules which set limits to health care that everyone can in principle accept. The result of such a contract might not be entirely different from the Nordic socialized medicine we know, but I believe that it will provide us with more sensible and more explicit guidelines to make health care more efficient, professional, just and—if solidarity means attending to the weakest and whose needs are greatest—more solidaristic.

NOTES

1. Matti Häyry, "European Values in Bioethics: Why, What and How to Be Used?" *Theoretical Medicine and Bioethics*, 24 (2003), p. 199.

2. Harry E. Emson, "Down the Oregon Trail—The Way for Canada?" *Canada Medical Association Journal*, 145:11 (1991), p. 1441.

3. Rob Houtepen and Ruud ter Meulen, "The Expectation(s) of Solidarity: Matters of Justice, Responsibility and Identity in the Reconstruction of the Health Care System," *Solidarity in Health Care,* eds. R. Houtepen and R. ter Meulen, *Health Care Analysis*, 8:4 (2000), p. 359.

4. *Cf.* Norman Daniels, *Just Health Care* (Cambridge: Cambridge University Press 1985), p. 141.

5. I refer to the following reports: *Priority-Setting in the Health Service* (Etisk Råd, Denmark 1996), *From Values to Choices* (STAKES, Finland 1995), *Priorities in Health Care* (SOU, Sweden 1995). There is an English summary in the Icelandic report *Forgangsröðun í heilbrigðismálum* (Icelandic Ministry of Health, 1998).

6. *Cf.* Will Kymlicka, *Contemporary Political Philosophy* (Oxford: Oxford University Press, 1990), p. 4.

7. *Priority-Setting in the Health Service*, p. 66.

8. *Priorities in Health Care*, p. 105.

9. *Priority-Setting in the Health Service*, p. 66.

10. *Choices in Health Care, Choices in Health Care*, A Report by the Government Committee (The Netherlands, 1992), p. 59.

11. Karl Marx, "Kritik des Gothaer Programms," *Die Neue Zeit*, 18 (1890–1891).

12. *Priority-Setting in the Health Service*, p. 105.

13. Eric Matthews, "Is Health Care a Need?" *Medicine, Health Care and Philosophy*, 1 (1998), pp. 156–157.

14. *Forgangsröðun í heilbrigðismálum*, p. 11.

15. *Priorities in Health Care*, p. 107.

16. Nicola Pasini and Massimo Reichlin, "Solidarity and the Role of the State in Italian Health Care," *Solidarity in Health Care*, p. 348.

17. *Ibid.*

18. John Rawls, *A Theory of Justice* (Oxford: Oxford University Press 1972), p. 12.

19. Kymlicka, *Contemporary Political Philosophy*, p. 62.

20. Tuija Takala, "Justice for All: The Scandinavian Approach," *Medicine and Social Justice*, eds. R. Rhodes, M. P. Battin and A. Silvers (Oxford: Oxford University Press 2002), pp. 184–185.

21. *Ibid.*, p. 189.

22. John Rawls, "Justice as Fairness: Political not Metaphysical," *Philosophy and Public Affairs*, 14:3 (1985), p. 231.

23. Houtepen and ter Meulen, "New Types of Solidarity in the European Welfare State," *Solidarity in Health Care.*

24. Jürgen Habermas, "Morality and Ethical Life: Does Hegel's Critique of Kant Apply to Discourse Ethics?" *Moral Consciousness and Communicative Action* (London: Polity Press, 1989), p. 200.

25. Susan Moller-Okin, "Reason and Feeling in Thinking about Justice," *Ethics*, 99:2 (1989), pp. 229–249.

26. Houtepen and ter Meulen, "The Expectation(s) of Solidarity," p. 373.

27. Daniels, *Just Health Care*.

28. *Ibid.*, *e.g.*, pp. 26 and 33.

29. Robert M. Veatch, *A Theory of Medical Ethics* (New York: Basic Books, 1981), chapter 11, "The Principle of Justice."

30. Daniels, *Just Health Care*.

31. Thomas McCarthy, "Kantian Constructivism and Reconstructivism: Rawls and Habermas in Dialogue," *Ethics*, 105 (1994), pp. 44–63.

Twelve

WILL YOU STILL NEED ME, WILL YOU STILL FEED ME, WHEN I'M 64? AN ETHICAL PROBLEM FOR THE MODERN, COSMOPOLITAN ACADEMIC

Søren Holm

People who deliberately abstain from having children do not make themselves responsible for the well-being of future generations. The question, then, is, can a duty of consideration be imposed on them by the weight of the parents' obligation toward their offspring? Is transferred parental responsibility legitimately enforceable?[1]

1. Introduction

The question raised by the Beatles in their 1967 Lennon and McCartney song is a question that must be of increasing interest to the modern, cosmopolitan academic, maybe not at the age of 64, given the increases in average life expectation, but for some later age (please note that the use of "cosmopolitan" here has no connection to the identification of "cosmopolitanism" as a left deviation from the party line in the Stalin era of the Soviet Union, nor to the title of a well known women's magazine).

Why is the question of interest? It is of interest because many of the traditional answers to who should need me and feed me when I am old, and I guess that for the Beatles' audience 64 was ancient, are under pressure. The pressure comes partly from changes in social conditions, partly from changes in policy emphasizing personal responsibility and partly from a change in emphasis in ethics towards more liberal ideas at the expense of communitarianism.

The social changes are mainly a reduction in family size with a resulting shrinking in the size and extension of the extended family and greater geographical mobility both within and between countries. This means that fewer people will have children who will feed them, fewer people will have nephews and nieces who might feed them, and more people will lose a strong connection with a locality or a country that might otherwise have generated a feeling of solidarity or obligation in those sharing the same locality or country. The cosmopolitan academic may therefore find that no one stands in one of those relationships to him or her that has traditionally been the basis for obligations to care for the aged.

Many medical technologies promise to be able to extend our lifespan and remove the diseases often afflicting old age, thereby leading to a long and healthy life, with no need to have anyone else than myself feed me at 64 or 84, although I might unfortunately have to work much longer before retirement. It is, however, unlikely that the more significant life expanding and morbidity compressing potential of these technologies will be ready for use before any of us who now contemplate 64 or 84 as actually approaching will reach those ages.

2. Is There an Obligation to Feed the Old?

This raises the question whether we can provide a philosophical argument for the existence of an obligation to feed the old? This is not an insurmountable problem if we are really talking about feeding or other very basic needs, but what about an obligation to ensure that the cosmopolitan academic has a tolerable old age with suitable access to wine, music and good food?

Within a liberal framework we might initially say that this problem should be solved by the person in question. At a young age each of us ought to make prudent choices ensuring that we can provide for ourselves in our old age (under reasonable assumptions about the future, for instance, life expectancy, needs in old age, and investment climate), either by having children and treating them so well that they will be obligated to support us, or by saving enough.

But the savings option does, although indirectly also rely on the continued "production" of children. Unless your savings are in the resources you actually need (say, food), long term savings in fungible assets (for instance, money) only keep their value in so far as there is an economic system in which some people continue producing sufficient, economically valuable outputs (please note that there is a distinction between what is valuable *sub specie aeternitatis* and what is economically valuable). If no one had children and the production base therefore gradually diminished the value of savings would also diminish.

A liberal response to the "when I am 64" question in terms of individual responsibility therefore only works if a sufficient number of children are born in each generation.

Some liberals, including Matti Häyry have argued that it is actually morally wrong to bring children into the world. Häyry writes:

I am convinced it is irrational to have children. This conviction is based on two beliefs that I hold. I believe it would be irrational to choose the course of action that can realistically lead to the worst possible outcome. And I believe that having a child can always realistically lead to the worst possible outcome, when the alternative is not to have a child.

I am also personally convinced that it is immoral to have children. Children can suffer, and I think it is wrong to bring about avoidable suffering. By deliberately having children parents enable suffering which could have been avoided by reproductive abstinence. This is why I believe that human procreation is fundamentally immoral.[2]

This creates a problem for the line of argument we have been pursuing above, especially if our cosmopolitan academics are also liberal philosophers. In that case they would have to argue either that the badness of procreation is outweighed in a consequentialist manner by the general benefits it produces, including the stabilizing effect on the value of savings, or that it is acceptable to benefit from other peoples' immoral actions (we can probably assume that the pleasurableness of sex and/or peoples'—on this line of argument—immoral desires to have children will mean that procreation will continue to occur). The second of these arguments, that it is acceptable to benefit from other peoples' immoral actions is not unproblematic. It clearly matters how one benefits, whether the immoral actions are past, present or future, whether the continuation of the benefit relies on the continuation of the immoral practice, and whether one is directly or indirectly condoning the immorality. The liberal self-sufficiency solution relies on continued procreation and it is difficult to see how our cosmopolitan academics must not at least tacitly condone this practice, as it is the only practice that can ensure them a tolerable old age. They are thus close to performative inconsistency. For those who are already 64 or are approaching this age in the not too distant future this is not a problem because we know that enough people have pursued reproduction in those 64 years to create a sufficient number of children to keep the economy running for the next many years. But for younger cosmopolitan liberals it is a real issue.

But can we do better in attempting to generate some obligation on others? The liberal can generate obligations in three ways: 1) by the free choice of individual agents, 2) by some sort of explicit, implicit or hypothetical contract, and 3) by positing human rights. I will here assume without further argument that the liberal can only unproblematically posit negative human rights and that a positive obligation to provide for other people in their old age (except as noted above to provide the bare minimum) cannot be generated through a liberal human rights approach, and therefore not discuss the third option any further.

The first liberal approach is not very promising. Some people will freely choose to commit themselves to helping some other people and will thereby choose to create an obligation to help them. But it is highly unlikely that a network of obligations produced in this way will extend to everyone who needs it, and because of their itinerant lifestyle the cosmopolitan academics may be in a particularly vulnerable position. Although we might consider bringing back a general academic version of that part of the Hippocratic Oath where the medical apprentice promises to:

> To hold him who has taught me this art as equal to my parents and to live my life in partnership with him, and if he is in need of money to give him a share of mine....[3]

It is, however questionable how effective such a promise would be. It is, for instance unlikely that most philosophy student would feel bound by it.

The second approach looks more promising, the literature abound with veil of ignorance arguments generating all sorts of obligations with excellent liberal, or at least Rawlsian, credentials, so why not an obligation to help people who have grown old. The old could perhaps even be conceptualized as the Rawlsian "least well of." I think that this is a possible line of argument, but it suffers from one general weakness and a specific problem. The weakness is the traditional weakness of all hypothetical contract arguments that it is unclear why actual people should be bound by hypothetical contracts. This weakness is especially acute when the veil of ignorance argument produces positive obligations that cannot be fully discharged individually. As an individual I cannot discharge an obligation to ensure that all old people are provided with sufficient resources to live a tolerable life (even if this obligation was circumscribed by jurisdiction or locality). It is an obligation that only WE can discharge through some kind of (re-)distributive social system. But what would be the argument for forcing me to contribute to this social system if, for instance I had no elderly relatives and I suffered from a disease that would strike me down in late middle age? After all the "patron saint" of liberal thinking John Stuart Mill famously held:

> that the sole end for which mankind are warranted, individually or collectively, in interfering with the liberty of action of any of their number, is self-protection. That the only purpose for which power can be rightly exercised over any member of a civilised community, against his will, is to prevent harm to others.[4]

Keeping my money in my pocket is presumably covered by the Millian "liberty of action," and the harm to others so remote and unspecific that it would infringe my liberty to extract the money from my pocket by force (e.g. by taxation).

The more specific problem is that the outcome of veil of ignorance arguments is crucially dependent on the specification of the original situation behind the veil and the stipulated properties of the veil. Who are the negotiators, what are the limits to the question they are discussing, and what information does the veil filter out? If the question is one about intergenerational justice are the negotiators only looking at obligations towards the elderly, or are they also looking at obligations toward the young? Do they know whether they live in an affluent or a poor society?

For a veil of ignorance argument to get off the ground we clearly need to specify the situation in some way, but all specifications are arbitrary to some degree and all already contain the outcome hidden in the specifications. It is therefore perhaps better to see veil of ignorance arguments as persuasive instead of justificatory. As a device we use to convince others that a given set of social rights and obligations are fair.

In the current context it seems excessively arbitrary to ask only one question along the lines of "would agents behind a veil of ignorance create an obligation to provide everyone with a tolerable old age?" without putting this in the complete context of inter- and intra-generational justice.

Given these problems with the highly hypothetical contracts generated by veil of ignorance arguments it might seem preferable to ask what contracts people would enter into from the positions they really possess in society (i.e. move to slightly less hypothetical, but still not actual contracts). If we can generate a definite answer to that question we can say to the non-compliant that this is really the contract they would have entered into in their full individuality, and that they therefore should feel bound by it. But we do again run into, perhaps even more intractable specification problems. Should we imagine the negotiation taking place between everybody at a certain stage in life (e.g. at the age of 18)? Does the negotiation cover everybody in society, or are there sub-contracts between specific groups (e.g. those who want to have children, smokers, religious people etc.) and who decides this question? Do we discuss each possible obligation in isolation (e.g. who has obligations towards children) or do we discuss the whole complex web of obligations between people (allowing for bargains between those with children and those without)? How do we deal with people moving between societies, like our cosmopolitan academics? This latter question becomes relevant because we are here discussing hypothetical contracts based on peoples' actual resource endowments, values and desires and we have every reason to believe that such contracts will differ significantly between societies (even if hypothetical contracts established behind a thick veil of ignorance might not differ to any great degree).

All of these specification problems indicate that it is problematic to engage in too tight specification, since the only purpose of that seems to be to be able to either to generate, or to rule out certain specific obligations. The bottom line is therefore that both our completely hypothetical veil of ignorance con-

tract and our slightly less hypothetical contract between actual people in affluent societies will probably incorporate an obligation to help people to have a
tolerable old age, whether they are cosmopolitan academics or not, but that
they will only do so as one part of a complicated web of obligations, many of
which the individual agent would not have chosen to be bound by if they were
negotiated separately, for instance an obligation to support the education of
other peoples' children.

If, however, it really is immoral to have children, even these kinds of argument will be in vain, since the obligation towards the elderly will never be
able to be discharged and they must die destitute (physician assisted suicide
always being an option for the liberal if any physician can be found young
enough to retain a license).

3. Conclusion

Who will feed the cosmopolitan academic at 64 (or 84)? Fortunately the question does not arise in its most acute form for cosmopolitan academics that are
now approaching that age. In the western world we live in societies where
most states have not yet fully realized the implications of philosophical liberalism (in both senses of "realize") and in which there are still a sufficient number of people having children to safeguard at least some of the value of our
savings (including importantly the value of our pension funds). Even in old age
we can therefore rely both on state enforced beneficence and on the continued
support of the economic system provided by our own, and other peoples' children.

For the liberal cosmopolitan academic it must be a very troubling state of
affairs to see ones old age supported by illiberal government policies and by
the immorality and folly of continued procreation, but maybe the deep sense of
unease this must engender can be relieved by a few glasses of red wine and the
words of the immortal Danish rock band Gasolin (played at a volume appropriate to overcome any hearing impairment caused by old age):

> Og Floridor ja
> og Celestin
> de siger hva' ska' du ha' min dreng
> jeg si'r det bedste
> til mig og mine venner, ja ja ja.

NOTES

1. Matti Häyry, "Is Transferred Parental Responsibility Legitimately Transferable?" Abstract, *XXIInd EACME Conference & XIXth European Conference on Philosophy of Medicine and Health Care*, August 24-27, 2005, p. 38.

2. Matti Häyry "A Rational Cure for Prereproductive Stress Syndrome," *Journal of Medical Ethics*, 30 (2004), p. 377.

3. Ludwig Edelstein, *The Hippocratic Oath: Text, Translation, and Interpretation* (Baltimore: Johns Hopkins Press, 1943).

4. John Stuart Mill, *Utilitarianism, On Liberty, and Considerations on Representative Government* (London: Dent, 1987), p. 78.

Part Four

TESTS AND EXPERIMENTS

Thirteen

UNIVERSAL RAPID TESTING FOR INFECTIOUS DISEASE IN AIRPORTS AND PLACES OF PUBLIC CONTACT: A THOUGHT EXPERIMENT ABOUT THE ETHICAL CHALLENGES

Margaret P. Battin, Charles B. Smith, Larry Reimer,
Jay A. Jacobson, and Leslie P. Francis

1. Introduction

New molecular technologies utilizing polymerase chain reactions, monoclonal antibodies, and recombinant antigens make possible rapid, inexpensive diagnosis of infectious disease in a fraction of earlier testing times. OraQuick, for example, identifies HIV-1 status with 99.3% sensitivity and 99.8% specificity[1] in just 20 minutes—down from the two-week test and confirmation test of earlier methods—and has high reliability whether a blood sample or oral fluid swab is used. Similar rapid tests are available or under development for many infectious diseases, including, for example, malaria, dengue, meningitis, SARS, and influenza. While molecular rapid tests vary in method, the emphasis is on speed, and most offer results in much less than an hour. But the prospect of widespread rapid testing by molecular methods also presents ethical challenges. Here, using a thought experiment, we want to explore the implications of rapid testing for infectious disease for such ethical concerns as liberty, privacy, confidentiality, consent, and justice and just procedure. Could a decent society agree to a policy of universal or near-universal rapid testing for infectious disease?

Rapid diagnosis has of course long been valuable in many areas of medicine, especially in infectious disease: the gram stain and rapid testing of throat cultures for strep are obvious examples. The trained eye of the experienced clinician has until recently been the fastest of all technologies, recognizing measles or the smallpox rash on the spot. It cannot, however, see everything, especially where contagiousness precedes visible symptoms, and the new rapid-test methods may mark both a dramatic technological advance and the

emergence of new ethical dilemmas. In the light of the extraordinary technological advance that rapid testing represents, we'd like to explore—in a specu-
lative way—just how far this advance could go if widely applied and still remain ethically acceptable.

The practical question is whether the new possibility of rapid, highly reliable testing might underwrite its near-universal use in public venues in an effort to lower—or eradicate—the global burden of infectious disease; the ethical question is whether this would so severely violate the basic norms of morality that it could not be tolerated. To be sure, the technologies imagined here
are not all now available—though some are—and it may never become possible to develop some of them; but we must also recognize that the thought experiment pursued here may be easily realizable in the near future.

2. A Thought Experiment: Rapid Testing at Airports
for Transmissible Infectious Disease

So consider a thought-experiment. Suppose that molecular rapid testing is
available for all known communicable infectious diseases, both those that involve human-to-human transmission and those that are transmitted via an intermediate vector. Testing for at least some conditions is no more invasive than
the collection of an oral fluid sample, easily accomplished with single cotton
swab rubbed inside the lip by a person with virtually no training. For others, a
simple pinprick for blood is all that is required. Whatever the samples, the new
rapid tests are more sensitive and specific than prior testing methods; let us
suppose that they are all as good as OraQuick is for HIV-1, with over 99%
sensitivity, nearly 100% specificity. There'll be a few cases missed, but virtually no false positives. Also imagine that test processing units are small, port-
able, and cheap enough so that they can be used in virtually any setting. Since
refrigeration, storage, running water, electricity, and sterile syringes are not
necessary, collection and testing can be performed virtually anywhere, in the
developed or developing world.

Anywhere? Imagine airports, for instance. Suppose, in this thought-
experiment, that as you check in at the Departures desk you supply, along with
your ticket and your passport or picture ID, an oral swab, quickly taken with
Q-tip supplied by the airline or a drop of blood from a tiny, sterile, automated
and virtually painless finger-prick, that is processed on the spot. Between the
time you check in and the time you arrive at the gate, your test is completed
and the result relayed by computer to the gate agents as well as to a national or
global disease-surveillance network that keeps track of the incidence of the
various infectious diseases. If you're "clean," you can board the plane. But if
you have TB or SARS or even just the flu, your test is repeated in another 20
minutes using an alternative assay if available (thus reducing the already low
probability of a false positive), and if the positive result is confirmed, you're

turned away, referred to the airport health clinic for whatever treatment is available. The same is true for the crew as well. You aren't singled out or profiled for risk; just as with baggage screening, everybody's tested. But nobody boards the plane unless they have a negative test result. In our thought-experiment, nobody boards the plane with a disease they could transmit to anybody else—at least, with one that has been identified through the rapid test procedure.

An intolerable invasion of liberty and privacy? A colossal inconvenience and disruption of people's plans? Violation of a basic liberty, the right to freedom of travel? An utterly unacceptable state-mandated invasion of the body? But consider what such a policy could prevent. Much of the most vivid public worry about the transmission of infectious disease, especially highly contagious emerging diseases like Ebola or SARS, involves intercontinental transmission that is only a single plane trip away. After all, HIV was originally believed to have arrived in San Francisco in 1981 with a single airline steward (though more recent evidence shows evidence of the virus in the U.S. several years earlier). In 2003, SARS arrived in Toronto from China in 2003 by plane: a 78 year old Scarborough grandmother, Kwan Sui Chu, contracted SARS at the Metropole Hotel in Hong Kong on February 21, 2003, and returned to Toronto two days later, where she infected her son; he entered Scarborough Grace Hospital, which would become the epicenter of the Toronto epidemic.[2]

Rapid testing at airports might have prevented both these occurrences of long-distance transmission of highly infectious diseases, and, assuming transmission would not have been repeated later in some other way, would have prevented some 44 SARS deaths in Toronto and thousands upon thousands of AIDS deaths in the U.S. alone. Keeping just a few passengers from boarding their planes, whoever they were, could have prevented huge loss of life.

Denying air travel to people with infectious diseases, as this thought-experiment would, isn't intended just to prevent passengers who might sneeze on their seatmates from giving a cold to others on board; in this thought-experiment, a state-mandated policy of this sort would prevent any person who is identified as a vector of disease from transmitting it later on in the place to which they intended to travel. Such a program would, we can assume, dramatically reduce the spread of infectious disease—not only that transmitted over long distances, like the Scarborough grandmother's unwitting transmittal of SARS from Hong Kong to Toronto, but that passed around at home, as she equally unwittingly infected her son.

3. Objections to the Thought Experiment's Universal-Testing Policy

There are many potential objections to this thought experiment. Here are four:

A. Violations of Liberty

Imagine the restrictions of liberty—not only the huge inconvenience, but the curtailment of freedom—multiplied by the millions of air passengers who would at one time or another be forced to stay behind. This might well seem to outweigh the gain in preventing the spread of disease: after all, intercontinental transmission of life-threatening potentially epidemic diseases, though it has occurred in cases like HIV and SARS, is comparatively rare. And some violations of liberty would have no basis: even if the new rapid-test technologies have lower false positive rates than the older, slower tests, if they are administered to huge numbers of passengers—indeed, all passengers and all crew on every flight, there may be some number of people mistakenly identified and kept behind.

Of course, false positives are hardly the problem, since, we assume, they would be comparatively few compared to true positives. The burden they impose, moreover, may be comparatively minor: brief delay until, with a 20-minute retest, the diagnosis is corrected. To be sure, air travelers might have to build in a few extra minutes to allow for the possibility of a retest, but this would not even be necessary if the testing process could be incorporated into the screening lines found at major international airports today. The real issue is whether identification of *true* positives in this way is an objective that can be ethically acceptable. After all, if rapid tests were routinely administered for all known infectious diseases, as we are supposing, there would be very substantial numbers of people correctly identified as infected by one or more disease-causing organisms. Disease-surveillance networks on a national or global scale, making accurate identification of outbreaks possible, would assemble huge amounts of data. To be sure, sophisticated forms of molecular testing might be able to distinguish between people in communicable phases of specific diseases, people in incubation phases but not yet contagious, people currently undergoing effective treatment for disease, or people who carry antibodies from former exposures but who can no longer transmit the disease. For this thought-experiment, however, assume just that it identifies anyone who could pass a disease along to someone else, either directly or through an intermediate vector. People testing positive would be detained and offered treatment, barred from their flights and other movement through check points—their liberty sharply curtailed—until no longer infected with a disease they could transmit.

But not everybody flies in planes. So continue the thought experiment: the rapid-test equipment, yielding results for (let us assume) all known communicable infectious diseases in just 20 minutes, can be used not only in airports but in schools, stadiums, hospitals, churches, movie theatres, shopping centers, even your local grocery store. Schools? Between the time you enter the vestibule and the time you're allowed to stuff your books in your locker, you are tested; it's straight to the school infirmary if you have a communicable disease. Hospitals? Nursing homes? Between the time you check in at the front desk and the time you're allowed to visit a friend or make rounds on your patients there, you're tested—whether you're a visitor or the physician. Riding the train or entering the subway? A short 20-minute delay would be all that's necessary before you're on your way—or held back, in the interests of keeping you from transmitting your disease to others, whether in the confined space of a public vehicle or to whatever contacts you might meet at your destination. The same picture could be true in the third world as in the first: there would be no entry into spaces of close human contact without first ensuring that you will not bring your transmissible disease with you. In many places—airports, schools, stadiums, tall buildings—you may already be screened for weapons, and some institutions—prisons and the military, for example—already do quite broad testing as one enters. Our thought experiment about universal infectious-disease testing is a screening of a related sort, in that it screens you for your potential to cause harm to others.

The magnitude of inconvenience and violations of liberty this thought experiment suggests may seem overwhelming. No easy freedom of movement, no spontaneous travel, no liberty of association—virtually all public movement and contact is potentially constricted in the interests of protecting others. Of course, not all movement and association is restricted—those who are disease-free can still board planes or go to the market or visit their (noninfectious) friends in hospitals, but if you are sick, you cannot pass through until you no longer test positive. As tests become available that can distinguish between persons who are infected and persons who are contagious, the restriction would need only to extend until the contagious period has passed.

To be sure, your inconvenience needn't always be great. For many diseases, point-of-care or over-the-counter tests can be used in advance, before you set out for the airport or other public place. Inconvenience and financial impact could be reduced: for example, airlines could be required not to penalize passengers by charging higher fares for those forced to change their departure dates in this way, and schools and workplaces required not to flunk students or dock workers with confirmed evidence of communicable disease. To be sure, not all costs can be avoided: there will be meetings and weddings missed, vacations cancelled, and reunions thwarted. For specific diseases with long-term transmission possibilities—HIV or TB, for instance—proof of ongoing treatment or perhaps an antibody titer could be provided, much as one requires a special permit to carry a gun aboard a plane. But the violation of liberty is often substantial: for diseases with acute phases and high transmission profiles—polio or influenza—you cannot pass through public spaces where testing is required until you are no longer identified as infected—or, more precisely, as contagious. No excuses and no exceptions: dignitaries and pilots are tested at the airport just as routinely as coach class passengers are, while ballplayers and their coaches are tested at the stadium just as routinely as the spectators and clergy and their altar attendants are tested at churches along with all their parishioners. In this thought-experiment, universal testing means just that—universal—in all places of public congregation and contact.

The financial costs of universal testing might be great, especially at the outset as people adjusted to the screening programs. The costs of disease avoided might be even greater, especially if screening programs were limited to more serious infectious diseases. Our question here concerns the moral costs of such a program.

B. Violations of Privacy and Confidentiality

Under this thought-experiment, state-mandated testing would be done just in places of public contact, as people move from one location to another. This would also raise substantial privacy and confidentiality issues. Suppose, for instance, you are denied boarding your flight but your partner is not: there may be a deeply embarrassing, now-public fact to explain. The only way you will be able to prevent the information that you have not passed the screening test (for whatever reason) from coming to light will be to avoid the test in the first place—that is, by not traveling in any public place. Of course, some privacy concerns about state-mandated testing do not arise: invading your home or your bedroom to catch you transmitting HIV or other STDs would not be necessary if carriers of such viruses are identified in routine public screening while you are out in the world somewhere; screening need not catch you in the transmission act. Violations of confidentiality could be minimized with strict controls on the nature of information reported to a national or global infectious-disease surveillance network. For example, if contact tracing is less necessary, surveillance data bases could be limited to data that are stripped of identifiers. Violations of confidentiality could also be limited by strict limits set on the uses to which surveillance information might be put. Yet privacy and confidentiality as well as liberty would be major concerns for an actual program of this sort, and the question is whether the ethical liabilities would be worth the gain.

C. Violations of Informed Consent and Just Procedure

Shades of Ellis Island? People with infectious diseases, after long and arduous sea-voyages in search of a better life, cut off at the border—inspected, barred from entry, held in involuntary quarantine, and shipped back where they came from, or, not infrequently, held in confinement until they died? Many if not most countries had such regulations, and they were all inhumane in the sense that they thwarted people's most basic dreams and consigned them to a public-health limbo or worse. The idea was to keep diseases out—tuberculosis, measles, diphtheria, trachoma, typhus, yellow fever, cholera, plague—and the only known way to do that was to keep the people who had these diseases out as well. Ships reporting cholera deaths were quarantined; for example, in the summer of 1892, the Hamburg-American liner *Moravia* arrived offshore at New York flying the yellow flag, reporting that 22 of 230 passengers had died of cholera during the voyage. Another 96 died during the following month, either on the way to New York or in quarantine.[3]

Exclusionary quarantine at national borders was practiced by many countries. For example, amid great public fear in the wake of the cholera epidemic of 1832, Canada established a quarantine station at Grosse Île, an island in the St. Lawrence 48 kilometers below Québec City, where ships with immigrants were required to land. By 1847, the migrations of poor and malnourished Irish fleeing the Great Famine were huge, with typhus and dysentery rampant among people packed in unsanitary conditions aboard ships unsuited for such large numbers. During the summer of 1847, some 5000 immigrants died at sea. Many more died waiting offshore for permission to land. Those who did land, some 12,000 immigrants, both sick and well, were held in quarantine on the island in grossly inadequate facilities. Many of those who had been well became ill, and many never reached their destination; 5424 are buried at Grosse Île.[4]

It is tempting to describe these events—now regarded as "one of the saddest pages in Canadian history"[5]—as an immense violation of justice, not only in trying to protect people on shore from disease but also as a response to public fears. Along with immigrants who were already ill, many others who were well were confined on ships or kept on Grosse Île, even when it was clear that they would become infected and die. These once-hopeful immigrants suffered and lived as *victims,* but they were perceived by the quarantine authorities— and particularly by the public—as *vectors.* These immigrants had hardly consented to such treatment; they had come to the New World for a better future, but were sent back, or died. This was not because they were trying to enter illegally or had past criminal records or for any other reason of policy-governed justice, but because some among them were discovered to have communicable infectious diseases—over which they had no control. They had no real opportunity for informed or voluntary consent before they sailed, and no guarantee of just procedure once they arrived. To be sure, some of this can be attributed to the huge numbers of immigrants that overwhelmed the border stations; but some of it was due to failure to recognize the ethical issues involved in treating people in these ways. Throughout history, quarantines, used by many authorities in many different time periods for many different diseases, may have reduced the extent of infectious-disease epidemics, even if they did not prevent them, but almost always at tremendous human cost.

Now consider our thought-experiment about molecular rapid testing in airports and other places of public contact. Is it as morally problematic as the crude border controls at Ellis Island, Grosse Île, and elsewhere around the world? The invasions and restrictions our thought-experiment posits may seem to be far greater: people who test positive for communicable disease cannot board planes, or trains, or ships, or for that matter even the downtown subway, whether in the developed or in the developing world. In the most far-reaching versions, assuming the relevant rapid-test technology can be devised that easily, quickly, cheaply, and accurately identifies those who could pass on infectious disease, not only cannot one visit a hospitalized friend, but one can be prevented from going to a ball game, shopping in a supermarket, going to church, going to one's class at school. This is a far more invasive conjecture than the kinds of border controls erected at Ellis Island or Grosse Île—those sieved out hundreds of boatloads of immigrant hopefuls, but this new conjecture would affect virtually *everybody.*

But therein lies the key. Ellis Island and Grosse Île's exclusionary policies had comparatively little effect and were clearly unjust because they were applied to new immigrants only—sometimes just to steerage-class passengers[6]—but did nothing to identify disease-carriers among people already in the country. They didn't work, or work sufficiently to avoid contagion overall, because they didn't affect *everybody.* In effect, some were forced to consent, while others were entirely excused. In no other situation were people already in the country screened in a universal and repeated way for infectious disease. True, there were extensive public health efforts to control infectious disease and heroic efforts to identify, treat, and prevent disease, but nothing that involved routine, regular, repeated screening of virtually the entire population. (Nor would it have been possible, since screening would have had to involve physical assessment by a physician or trained public-health official, not a simple sample read cheaply and automatically in 20 minutes or less.)

Thus the high moral cost of the exclusionary quarantine policies at Ellis Island, Grosse Île, and many other places around the world did not weigh well against these policies' effect in reducing the burden of disease. The idea in the thought-experiment we are considering here cuts the other way: these policies would sometimes involve moderate practical and moral costs—imposing restrictions of liberty, violations of privacy and confidentiality, and violations of requirements of informed consent (all perhaps involved in being forced to miss a plane)—but would promise huge public gains in reducing the burden of disease. But this does not yet entail that the ethical violation is warranted for the end in sight.

D. Violations of Justice.

It might also be said that universal screening of the sort our thought-experiment imagines, carried out on a global scale, would raise issues of distributive justice: since infectious disease is more prevalent among those of lower socioeconomic status and those in resource-poor countries, the moral costs of inconvenience and limitations of liberty, violations of privacy and confidentiality, and the burdens of coercion, would fall more heavily on already disadvantaged people. This would be injustice in the distribution of burdens, not benefits, but injustice just the same. However, this would be true just if, as on ships quarantined in New York harbor or waiting to land at the overwhelmingly crowded quarantine station at Grosse Île, people with serious or potentially fatal infectious diseases were left untreated and, as in that case, essentially left to die. On the contrary, this thought-experiment imagines that those identified with positive tests would not only have the advantage of diagnosis for conditions they might not have recognized, but would be guaranteed access to effective treatment as well.

This distributive picture is actually enhanced in our thought experiment by compensation for the least well off. There is a substantial benefit here, offsetting the nuisance value of routine testing and the occasional major inconvenience if one tests positive: you get a diagnosis of a disease you may not have known you had and with it, let us also assume, immediate treatment. This is a practical benefit, in avoiding the harms of disease, but it is a moral benefit too, in that it treats the person who tests positive not just as a *vector* and thus a risk to others, but as a *victim* as well, a human person in need of and deserving of help. It is a distributive benefit for groups of the least well off, those characteristically most burdened by ill health, and especially by infectious disease. If cheap, rapid, noninvasive testing of high reliability were used in virtually every public circumstance, from airports to schools to public transportation, accompanied by immediate treatment, it would mean inconvenience and real limitation for some time as well as substantial short-term societal expense, but its end result would be to detect and treat many or all forms of human-to-human communicable disease and much of that transmitted through intermediate vectors as well, thus virtually eliminating disease and hence improving the lives of all—especially the least well off.

To be sure, this outcome assumes that treatment exists for any infectious disease identified, that the treatment is effective, and that the treatment doesn't have serious side effects that might lead a person to refuse it. It also assumes that there won't be substantial numbers of people with other reasons for refusing treatment, such as religious convictions, but we leave that issue aside for now. The likelihood of meeting these assumptions may currently seem less than the likelihood of having the rapid-diagnosis tests, but let us assume for the purposes of this thought-experiment that effective therapy does exist.

Universal, free, effective treatment would be crucial if a program of universal testing is to achieve its goal, the virtually complete eradication of human-host-only infectious disease. With this guarantee, the poor, rather than being more greatly disadvantaged by such a scheme, would be its greatest beneficiaries: it is from their shoulders that the burden of infectious disease would be primarily lifted.

4. Underlying Conceptions of the Individual

These objections to the thought experiment about violations of liberty, about privacy and confidentiality, about informed consent, and about justice are to some degree all framed in the individualist conceptions of liberal theory, in which what is central is recognition of and respect for individual autonomy. But that very picture becomes problematic when we consider the biological realities of infectious disease. Elsewhere, we argue that in order to fully understand the moral challenge at hand, we must move beyond a conception of the individual seen as discrete and autonomous toward a conception that sees persons as relational and embodied—large organisms carrying and inhabited by a sea of tiny organisms that move in ways often beyond our control to other persons around us, as theirs do to us in turn.[7] To change this human situation and extricate ourselves from the web of mutual transmission in which we are caught, we must first revise—not scrap, but enhance—this underlying picture of ourselves. While we cannot fully explore this conceptual shift here, our thought experiment is intended to challenge traditional conceptions of the human individual and the moral principles that should govern how people treat each other.

What we need to do, in exploring the way in which these issues will reframe themselves in a modified view of autonomy as relational and embodied, is recognize that we—each "individual" agent—all have a *joint* interest in extricating ourselves from the web of mutual transmission of infectious disease. Under the traditional understandings of autonomy, an individual's objections may override invasions of liberty or the use of coercion, especially where some individuals are used for the advantage of others; under our modified account, the balance may well tip the other way, seeing even an invasive and coercive strategy like universal rapid-testing at points of public transport and contact as a legitimate measure to change the human condition of victimhood and vectorhood, threat and threatenedness, in infectious disease.

5. The Thought Experiment: A "Decade of Infectious-Disease Inconvenience"?

Call the period our thought-conjecture envisions the *"decade of infectious-disease inconvenience."* It's a considerable leap to be sure, but let us suppose that if this policy were in force for a decade, the frequency of positives would decline, presumably increasingly rapidly as disease was no longer being transmitted, and—as clearly detected by global disease-surveillance networks—eventually disappear. Like smallpox, not just one communicable disease but

all of them (or at least all of them without sizeable animal reservoirs not need-
ing transmission from humans) could be wiped from the face of the earth. At
the end of the decade, let us suppose, the entire apparatus of universal testing
could be dismantled and suspended, kept in readiness and only reinstituted if
some unanticipated outbreak were to occur.

Of course, such a policy would be ethically tolerable only under at least
these conditions:

1) the policy uses minimally restrictive alternatives, including the least
possible inconvenience and restraint of liberty;

2) invasion of privacy is minimized by discreetness in collecting samples
and confidentiality by permitting no other use, except for epidemiological
tracking, of test information;

3) discomfort and bodily invasion produced by the collection of samples
for the test is minimized and subjects are adequately informed about the
procedure being performed; and

4) adequate and immediate treatment is guaranteed for all those who do
test positive.

Could a decent society agree to a policy of near-universal rapid testing for
communicable infectious disease, one that might mean substantial restrictions
on some people for some time? Would a decent society also guarantee treatment for people testing positive for infectious disease? Even more, would a
decent society require treatment (or isolation) for those who did not want to
accept treatment, whether for religious reasons, fear of treatment, or to avoid
the side effects of treatment? No doubt actual social acceptance or rejection of
such policies would be a function of fear: if no threat were apparent at the
moment, testing and treatment policies would be resisted, but in or after an
outbreak of some disease that is widely feared, like SARS, Ebola, or person-
to-person avian flu, such measures might be widely embraced. Mandated
treatment might remain more controversial, but universal testing might be
quite likely to be embraced, much as airport screenings were embraced in the
wake of airliner hijackings—even though a good bit of grumbling about the
inconvenience might remain, yet little disagreement about the principle involved.

In theory, at least, just as with immunization for diseases, like smallpox,
that have been effectively controlled, immunization for further infectious diseases would eventually no longer be required. In principle, a resolute period of
universal rapid testing coupled with treatment for infectious diseases would
have the eventual effect of eliminating these diseases and thereby eliminating

the need for further such testing as well. To be sure, the possibility of complete disease eradication is greatest where the human is the only host—as in small-pox and polio, though not in some other serious infectious diseases—though the list of human-host-only diseases is nevertheless quite long, and similar testing regimens could be introduced for at least animal populations kept in controlled conditions, like poultry and cattle. A universal rapid-testing policy would be self-limiting in the end, as the various diseases were controlled and finally wiped out. Thus the invasions of liberty, privacy and confidentiality, informed consent, and justice generally involved in this policy would be temporary, short-lived, but its gains in the elimination of disease permanent. Perhaps simplistic ways of thinking about these moral issues would be put to rest as well: the individualist picture of one person's interests pitted against, rather than with, those of another, would need reform, and a revised understanding of the sense in which one individual's interests in liberty, privacy, confidentiality, and justice are violated would need to be developed. This would be a new ethical picture, perhaps an ancient dream of public health but new to bioethics—of individuals' common interest in extricating oneself—indeed, all of ourselves—from the web of infectious disease all human beings share.

Is this speculation a proposal, a thought-experiment, or what? Clearly, it isn't science fiction, or only science fiction: already, a research group headed by Dr. Paul Yager at the University of Washington is working under a $15.4 million Grand Challenges in Global Health grant from the Bill and Melinda Gates Foundation to develop diagnostic tools that can be more easily used in the developing world; their point-of-care diagnostic system anticipates being able to test blood for a range of diseases, including bacterial infections, nutritional status, and HIV-related illnesses. The investigators envision that health care workers would load a small blood sample onto a disposable test card about the size of a credit card, containing all of the necessary test re-agents; the test card would then be inserted into a device about the size of a handheld computer; it would yield results in about 10 minutes.[8] They don't, we believe, have universal airport screening for infectious disease in mind, but better diagnosis of multiple conditions in the developing world. Yet we can see the implications of technological developments such as this for the world as a whole, particularly as it confronts the threats of infectious disease. Would the developed world cooperate in the control of infectious disease as well?

Thus, in the end, this speculation isn't just a proposal or a thought-experiment; rather, it's an invitation to consider what price we would pay if we had some realistic chance of eliminating infectious disease—which, perhaps, we do: a *decade of infectious-disease inconvenience,* we might imagine, for the goal of virtually complete eradication. There'd be disagreement over the politics of such a program, of course, and especially over whether treatment would be mandated or measures like quarantine or isolation would be imposed on those who tested positive but refused available, effective treatment, but the challenge for us here is to consider the deeper ethical issues and the basis on which they rest. The very notion of "a price to pay" in terms of autonomy, restrictions of liberty, violations of privacy and confidentiality, and violations of justice suggests a conception of the individual and personal autonomy still seen as discrete, not yet fully understood as relational and embodied. To recognize that the ethical challenges raised here by our thought experiment are not in the end unethical, we must revise that underlying picture of ourselves that sees our interests as in competition rather than in concert in the control of transmission in infectious disease. Rather, our interests in this matter fortunately coincide, and we would all have a common interest in accepting rapid testing everywhere—airports and places of public contact—if we could thus rid ourselves of the universal burden of communicable infectious disease.

ACKNOWLEDGEMENT

A later version of this chapter has appeared under the title "A Thought Experiment: Rapid-Test Screening for Infectious Disease in Airports and Places of Public Contact" as chapter 15 of Margaret P. Battin, Leslie P. Francis, Jay A. Jacobson, and Charles B. Smith, *The Patient as Victim and Vector: Ethics and Infectious Disease* (New York: Oxford University Press, 2009).

NOTES

1. *Cf.* Alexi A. Wright and Ingrid T. Katz, "Home Testing for HIV," *New England Journal of Medicine*, 354:437-440 (2 February 2006), p. 4.
2. Philip W. H. Peng, David T. Wong, David Bevan, and Michael Gardam, "Infectious Control and Anaesthesia: Lessons Learned from the Toronto SARS Outbreak," *Canadian Journal of Anesthesia* 50:989-997 (2003), p. 2; *Toronto Star*, www.thestar.com/static/PDF/030926_sars_h4_h5.pdf, accessed 3.23.06.
3. "How We Guard Against the Introduction of Cholera: Where the Scourge Originated and How the Government Copes With It When It Gets to These Shores: Dr. Doty Explodes Some Erroneous Beliefs on the Subject of the Dread Disease." *The New York Times*, July 23, 1911, page 1, Sunday magazine section.
4. www.pc.gc.ca/lhn-nhs/qc/grosseile/docs/plan1/sec3/page2biii_E.asp, accessed 3.23.06.
5. www.pc.gc.ca/lhn-nhs/qc/grosseile/docs/plan1/sec3/page2bi_E.asp, accessed 3.23.06.
6. *New York Times,* July 23, 1911.
7. Margaret P. Battin, Leslie P. Francis, Jay A. Jacobson, and Charles B. Smith, *The Patient as Victim and Vector: Ethical Issues in Infectious Disease* (New York: Oxford University Press, 2009).
8. Bill and Melinda Gates Foundation, Grand Challenges in Global Health, project #14. http://www.gcgh.org/subcontent.aspx?SecID=391.

Fourteen

PIGS AND PRINCIPLES:
THE USE OF ANIMALS IN RESEARCH

John Harris

1. Introduction

My current interest in the ethics of human interactions with animals is partly the fault of Matti Häyry. I have for a long time been intrigued by his refusal to eat pork or indeed use pig derived products while himself remaining a meat eater. I have known and been impressed by Matti for more years than I care to admit. On first acquaintance I was struck by his intellectual honesty and ability to decline all compromise when it comes to issues of principle and his facility for articulating complex ideas in a clear and accessible manner. This combined with the driest of dry senses of humor and a capacity for enjoyment of life second-to-none, makes him a formidable companion and colleague and positively frightening at conferences, particularly after midnight! Matti, as he himself would be the first to agree, is not really old enough for a festschrift! The advantage however of being celebrated in this way at his comparatively early age is of course that there will be room for thee or four further volumes while he is still young enough to appreciate them.

I take as my point of departure for this essay Matti's provocative stance on the pig. Prompted by this and by the challenge it posed to me to think again about my approach to human interactions with animals, I looked for inspiration in the recent Nuffield Council on Bioethics report on the ethics of involving animals in research.[1]

The Nuffield Council set out to resolve the question of the ethics, the legitimacy, of using animals in research. If the use of animals is legitimate then it is obviously not simply sensible, but also perhaps mandatory to use animals in research. In particular to make the best estimates possible based on the effect on appropriate animal models of how substances and procedures will affect humans and in particular as to whether these substances or procedures are safe for human use. We humans also stand to learn much about animals and ourselves from this research including much that may be of use to animals. Many beneficial procedures for animals themselves have been developed from animal research. For all these reasons if we can ethically use animals for research there are powerful reasons why we should. But can we, and how are we to think about whether or not we can?

Of course the legitimacy of using animals in research partly depends on whether or not their use is necessary to protect human lives and interests and to promote human welfare. However such use might be ruled out from the start if there were compelling reasons to think that animals, or some animals, have the same rights and interests as humans or some humans, or rights and interests of similar nature and force to those which in normal circumstances protect most humans. We cannot after all (except perhaps in the most dire emergency) use some humans for the benefit of others without their consent. And indeed often we cannot use humans instrumentally even with their consent, as for example in the prohibition of the donation of vital organs (organs without which humans will die) for live donation. We do not permit competent humans to donate a heart for example.[2] We should now examine the Nuffield Council's considered answers to these questions.

2. The Nuffield Council Report (NCR)

The Nuffield Council devotes Chapters 3, 14 and 15 to ethical issues. The main conclusions are stated at paragraph 3.78:

> This chapter has aimed to lay out the critical elements of the current moral debate. We have argued that the following questions must be considered:
>
> i) The debate is not best characterised in terms of the relative moral status of humans and animals but in terms of what features of humans and animals are of moral concern, in the sense of making certain forms of treatment morally problematic.
> ii) Once those features are identified, the question needs to be asked as to how they should be taken into account in moral reasoning. Are they factors to be weighed against others, or do they function as absolute prohibitions?
> iii) Finally, what does it mean to be a moral agent? How should moral agency be considered in the regulatory framework that governs animal research?
>
> In general we have not attempted to provide answers to these questions at this stage. We invite readers to reflect upon the discussion and examples provided in the following chapters in an unbiased way, and in the light of their own conclusions thus far. We present the conclusions of the working Party in Chapters 14 and 15.

Turning to Chapter 14 we find conclusions in the form of 4 positions that might be taken on animal research, two of which are self-explanatory: The "anything goes" view, the "on balance justification" view (research is on balance justified), "moral dilemma" view, (either we wrong animals by experimenting or wrong humans by failing to do so) and the "abolitionist" view. The NCR opts for a "process" approach. This is summed up in paragraph 14.62:

> [A]lthough full substantive consensus may be unattainable, we conclude that there is genuine overlapping consensus in terms of process. Even if proponents of the "anything goes" view and the "abolitionist" view differ on the letter of the law … most reasonable proponents of both views are likely to accept that for so long as animal research continues, animals involved must be protected. It can be argued that in these circumstances a detailed system of licensing and inspection is a necessary and legitimate instrument to reconcile the different views that stakeholders and members of society hold.

This seems a useful and productive "solution" if we accept that agreement between the most radically opposed positions is unlikely, and that therefore some solution that builds on the fact of disagreement is the best that can be obtained.

However it also assumes that the extreme pro-animal view none-the-less accepts a difference in moral status between animals and humans or that the extreme pro-animal view is unreasonable. For if it were to be considered reasonable to regard animals as entitled to the same protections as humans, or likewise if it was reasonable to believe animals and humans shared the same moral status, then inviting those who share these views to accept animal research with protections would be like asking fellow citizens to accept or even participate in the "protected" murder or imprisonment and torture of other moral equals. But if there is a difference in moral status between animals and humans or, if the pro-animal view that denied this is demonstrably unreasonable, then the reasons for either of these conclusions would (probably) provide a basis for a definitive account of what is or is not morally permissible by way of animal research and use by humans and the process "solution" would be redundant.

Two further considerations are then discussed by Nuffield, they are the issues of "moral status" and "consistency."

3. Moral Status

I should myself declare an interest at this point, and it is that I have over many years developed and used a moral status account of personhood[3] which I believe helps both with distinctions between different human individuals (zygotes, embryos, neonates, and individuals in permanent vegetative state among others). As we have noted NCR rejects moral status as a helpful approach.

If the NCR is right when it claims that the "debate is not best characterized in terms of the relative moral status of humans and animals but in terms of what features of humans and animals are of moral concern, in the sense of making certain forms of treatment morally problematic" then only if animal research is unacceptable can moral status be irrelevant. Consider, three main features that are relevant to moral concern for animals are their capacity to feel pain, and experience suffering and premature death. The only way that pain, suffering or premature death of animals can be justifiable to spare humans the same, is either by establishing that pain, suffering and premature death are less bad, or less important when experienced by animals, or that even if they are qualitatively comparable (whatever that may mean), human interests are more important. Either or both of these considerations lead inexorably to a difference in moral status as the ground for permitting animals to be used instrumentally in the service of humans. More detail as to why this is so will emerge as we discuss moral status in more detail.

Thus, so far from it being true that the debate is "not best characterized in terms of the relative moral status of humans and animals," by far the best candidate for an explanation of the difference between most animals and most humans which might bear upon the legitimacy of the human use of animals is the idea of "moral status" and in the reasons for according that status. Moreover, as we have noted, the NCR establishes just this point only, perhaps inadvertently, to resile from it. It is moral status (or strictly the reasons for differences in moral status) that explains differences in ways in which it may be considered appropriate to treat certain individuals or classes of individuals and we follow the NCR definition of moral status in expanding on this point.

In the United Kingdom experimentation on human embryos is permissible, legal and widely accepted. Equally abortion, in some circumstances right up to term, is also legal and again widely accepted. These facts show that the human individual at certain stages has a different moral and legal status to that of normal adult humans for example.

These differences in moral and legal status are accepted in most jurisdictions and have been repeatedly upheld in the European Court of Human Rights.[4]

The NCR offers one major reason for rejecting the pivotal role of moral status; it is perhaps over-concentration on this point that leads NCR to sideline the idea of moral status which it elsewhere uses to good effect:

3.21 It could easily be assumed that the justification for using animals for research (and other uses) depends entirely on the question of the relative moral status of humans and animals. Then the defence of animal use would be the same task as showing that only humans have moral status, or that their status is in some way "higher" than that of animals. But this assumption might be too simplistic. Suppose it was possible to establish that … all humans are more important moral subjects than all animals. Yet this is not enough to show that animals can properly be sacrificed for human purposes. For it may be that although humans are morally more important than animals, they have a moral duty of *stewardship* to "lesser" beings ….

Therefore, the permissibility of harmful animal research does not follow by necessity from the assumption that humans have a higher moral status than animals.

While this last point about the permissibility of harmful research not following "by necessity" from moral status is surely right, it does not succeed in its purpose of demonstrating the irrelevance of moral status to the question of how animals can be treated. It is if course true that differences in moral status between most humans and most animals do not do all the work in justifying particular uses (or abuses) of animals. However, the reasons for differences in moral status can (and do usually) also show why human interests take priority over those of animals.

The concept of "stewardship" does not show that this moral status approach is sometimes false. Stewardship may be an obligation with respect to animals, but stewardship may imply duties to species or particular populations rather than to individuals or it may license the sacrifice of some individuals for the sake of others. Such forms of stewardship are not possible among humans precisely because we share a moral status which precludes the sacrifice of some innocent human individuals for the sake of others. (There are exceptional circumstances in which such trade-offs between human lives are made and condoned, but almost all moral theories and the political and legal systems of all democratic societies combine to identify such trade-offs as unethical and illegal.) Stewardship of animals by humans may therefore be consistent with population management which may involve culling and other selective killing of individuals, principally because we humans are satisfied that animals have a different moral status which does not preclude such forms of stewardship. If you can sacrifice individual animals to animal populations, or indeed some individuals for the benefit of other individual animals, then it is less difficult to justify their sacrifice for human populations (by hypothesis populations of a more important moral status). The contrary is also false. We humans often regard ourselves as in some sense stewards of one another, but again, contra the way stewardship is perceived and is justifiable in the case of animals, this does not imply that selective culling (even if demonstrably in the interests of the species) is ever justifiable.

We note that there are of course justifications available for killing and otherwise harming creatures of the same moral status as ourselves: killing in war and in self-defense, imprisonment of criminals and so on are all done to other people who share our moral status, they are all equally the bearers of rights with important interests we are normally obliged to respect. However the difference in moral status between humans and animals usually reflects the defensible belief that animals lack important rights and interests which, if present, would afford protection from being killed or harmed except in pursuit of a just war, self-defense etc.[5]

Equally, while the difference in moral status may not straightforwardly license the infliction of pain on animals, if important differences in moral status are sustainable, this does imply important differences in how the legal and moral doctrine of "necessity" is to be understood between creatures of different moral status, so that we may the more easily imagine and justify the necessity of using creatures of lesser rather than those of greater moral status.

4. Consistency

In Chapter 15 the NCR sets out its main conclusions. Paragraph 15.9 states emphatically:

> All research licensed in the UK has the potential to cause pain, suffering, distress or lasting harm to the animals used. Most animals are killed at the end of experiments. A world in which the important benefits of such research could be achieved without causing pain, suffering, distress, lasting harm or death to animals involved in research must be the ultimate goal.

This is a daring and radical conclusion, for while all would agree to the aim of eliminating "pain, suffering, distress," and "lasting harm," the addition of "death" to this list raises acute issues of consistency. It invites readers of NCR to endorse the principal of accepting as an ultimate goal a world in which "the important benefits of such research could be achieved without causing ... death" to animals. It is difficult to see how if there are ethical considerations which mandate this as the goal for animal research it should not also be the goal for all human interactions with animals including food production and sport. While all would agree to the aim of eliminating *pain, suffering, distress*, and *lasting harm*, the addition of *death* to this list is highly problematic. Why should this be the goal of all research in the UK when it is not the goal of all food production or of all use of working animals or of animals in sport? Indeed it is not even on the agenda of all food production let alone national policy on food production. There is a real issue here for science as to whether the elimination of all animal research is an appropriate goal for science even as an ideal? It may be both wrong in principle and indeed unnecessary for science to embrace the objective of eradicating research on animals, when the killing of animals for more trivial purposes is neither the objective of most individuals, nor of most religions, nor of most moral systems, nor of most political parties or movements nor of most societies which undertake science research. Of course if the killing of animals is clearly a moral wrong, there is not only no reason why science should not take a lead here, there are some good reasons why it should. However not only is this far from established as a universally accepted moral objective (or even as an objective held by a significant minority) it seems far from being a realistic or urgent moral objective.

This is perhaps the time for a general investigation into the relations, moral political social commercial and scientific that obtain between humans and animals.

Given the numbers of animals involved the use of animals in research is a tiny proportion of the animals used and often killed for other human purposes and indeed for the purposes of other animals. The following passage from the NCR is particularly illuminating:

> [T]he view might be taken that the use of approximately 2.7 million animals in research is relatively insignificant when compared to more than 950 million livestock and nearly 500,000 tonnes of fish used annually for food production in the U.K. ... or when compared to the number of wild birds and mice killed by pet cats, which has been estimated to be 300 million per year.[6] The benefit to humans in using animals as food entails primarily an increased range in dietary variety, while the benefits of animal research can consist in significant developments in scientific progress and human welfare.

In view of these facts it is either odd, or perhaps evidence of terminal irrationality, that militant animal rights activists have targeted the scientific community rather than the food industry or domestic cats. (Indeed if domestic cats became the prime source of animals for research this might so to speak kill two birds with one stone.) It is perhaps a sad reflection on our society that scientists have so far commanded less public sympathy than would I am sure have been given to domestic cats (or indeed to the purveyors and consumers of burgers and bacon sandwiches) had they been the victims of the sustained campaign of violence and vilification that has been directed towards those involved in animal research.

This chapter has not attempted to resolve the question of the legitimacy of animal research. What it has done is indicate that the ethics of animal research will be resolved, if at all, by an account of moral status which can show whether or not animals or some animals can share the same moral status with humans or with some humans. In short whether animals or some animals can possess rights and/or interests which protect them from instrumentalization in the service of other creatures. It is difficult to see how the ethics of animal research or indeed of other uses of animals can be adequately addressed in the absence of general agreement on moral status.

We have also seen that it would be inconsistent to place limitations on the use of animals in science research which are not placed on the necessarily less urgent and morally important use of animals in food, sport, domestic service and farming.

NOTES

1. The Nuffield Council on Bioethics, *The Ethics of Research Involving Animals* (London: The Nuffield Council on Bioethics, 2005).

2. *Cf.* John Harris *Wonderwoman and Superman* (Oxford: Oxford University Press, 1992), chapters 5 and 6.

3. See John Harris, *Violence and Responsibility* (London: Routledge and Kegan Paul, 1980); John Harris *The Value of Life* (London: Routledge, 1985).

4. The European Court of Human Rights Case of Vo v. France (Application no. 53924/00) Strasbourg 8th July 2004. See also Case of Evans v. The United Kingdom (Application no. 6339/05), 7 March 2006; *cf.* Amel Alghrani, "Deciding the Fate of Frozen Embryos," *Medical Law Review*, 13:1 (2005), pp. 244-256.

5. See Harris, *The Value of Life*; Mary Ann Warren, *Moral Status* (Oxford: Clarendon Press, 1997); Robert A. Hinde, *Why Good is Good* (London and New York: Routledge, 2002).

6. The Nuffield Council on Bioethics, p. 27.

Fifteen

RESEARCH ETHICS: A DECENT PROPOSAL

Rosamond Rhodes

1. Introduction

Since I first met Matti Häyry, criticism has been an important and delightful feature of our interaction. In public meetings, in publications, in face to face conversations, and in email communications, I have learned from, and taken pleasure in, Matti's quick wit and insightful comments. Aside from these public and private bits of repartée, I have become a strong admirer of Matti's distinctive style of argument. The Häyry papers that I have enjoyed most make people rethink their positions and assumptions by challenging them with creative (counter-) examples. His paper, "A rational cure for pre-reproductive stress syndrome,"[1] is a case in point that also illustrates the Häyry brand of sarcasm. In that article Matti explains that the death of some embryos is frequently an inevitable consequence of reproductive activities because a significant percentage of the embryos that are created can then be expected to die. The foreseeable death of embryos from attempts at reproduction can, however, easily be prevented by abstaining from procreative activities. Hence, Häyry argues, those who see killing an embryo as murder are committed to avoiding procreative activities entirely. The only way to avoid Häyry's compelling conclusion is to give up one of premises as untenable, which I presume is the intended consequence of the extended discussion.

Häyry is superb at this form of argument, and he is clearly a master of making philosophy fun. For that reason, I take Matti to be a role model to those of us who see education and correction as important goals of our work in bioethics. In that light, Matti's work brings bioethics into the Socratic tradition.

I shall, therefore, take my task in this chapter to be honoring Matti as a true disciple of Socrates. He has enlightened me about issues in bioethics and showed me how to effectively bring humor and persuasive argument to bear in teaching sensitive and complicated material. I hope to repay that debt in kind.

In his comments on an early draft of a recent paper that I published on research ethics,[2] Matti suggested that I reverse the order of argument by starting, rather than ending, with my controversial example. He thought that the project would be clearer if I first put forward the example, and then went on to show why what I was suggesting was perfectly reasonable. At the time, I thought that reworking the paper as he suggested, would involve too much work and that it would also make people too indignant to take my arguments seriously. So, I did the paper my way. Readers were irate none the less and many failed to understand the substance of my position. I know this to be a fact because the paper received a surprisingly large amount of criticism, most of which showed significant misunderstanding of the view that I intended to put forth and seemed largely to miss my point. So, in this paper, I should like to try the argument again, but this time, doing it Matti's way.

It is also hard to pass up an opportunity to continue an ongoing argument with Matti Häyry. From his extensive work on utilitarianism it is clear that Häyry is a utilitarian with a particularly strong commitment to Mill's views on liberty.[3] From all that I have read I conclude that Häyry shares Mill's views on the importance of liberty and that he sees "the harm principle" as the singular justification for limiting liberty. In what follows, I also want to take issue with Matti on that position and press for accepting a broader range of reasons as justifying restrictions on liberty. We have previously jousted over this particular issue in the context of genetic ignorance[4] and abortion,[5] and now we can do it again in the context of research ethics.

2. A Decent Proposal for the Conduct of Human Subject Research in a Just Society

Imagine a just democratic state in which all residents have access to a national healthcare system that provides for treatment based on need and efficacy and that makes allocation decisions by employing broadly endorsed principles that are fairly applied. Further imagine that those residing in the state are largely satisfied with the national health system, its arrangements for the delivery of state of the art care, and its provisions for the timely and fair adjudication of disputes that arise from time to time.

In that same society now imagine that after sharing information about the conduct of human subject research (for instance, about actual harms that have been suffered by research subjects since the institution of research regulations, about advances achieved through previous studies and about options for improved research oversight), after an opportunity for discussion, and a period of lively free and open debate, a social consensus emerges and with bi-partisan support the legislature passes a bill that requires every resident to perform some research service, say, every ten years. According to the carefully crafted measure, while every one would be required to serve as a subject in some research study, each individual (or in the case of incompetent people, their surrogate decision maker) would be left the freedom to choose the particular project for research service from among all of the projects listed on a national web-site for which they meet the selection criteria. For healthy individuals, the

research participation obligation would be fulfilled by serving as a healthy subject or control. For individuals who required medical treatment or surveillance,
the research participation requirement could be fulfilled by accepting treatment
in the context of a study. Under this novel model, standard of care and innovative medical treatment that still involved areas of uncertainty would frequently
be deemed simultaneously as both research and treatment, and patients would
be encouraged to accept the role of study subjects in ongoing investigations of
intervention efficacy and complications.

3. Arguments for Instituting this Proposal

Because this society and this proposal are only imagined, I cannot actually
recount the arguments that led to its adoption. I can only provide the kind of
arguments that would lead to such a conclusion and offer a rebuttal for the
kinds of objections that readers are likely to raise.

Since World War II, we have witnessed a dramatic increase in biomedical
knowledge and tremendous progress in creating effective treatments for disease. These are benefits that flow from human subject research. We are also
aware that we stand on the brink of a cascade of spectacular advances in biomedical technology related to insights into human genetics, the promise of
stem cell research, and the growing understanding of the role of viruses in diseases such as cancer and the possibility of preventing them through immunization. Developments in genetic screening, genetic testing, pharmaco-genetics
(which would match drugs with individuals based on the individual's genetic
likelihood of responding) and gene-transfer therapy as well as tissue replace-
ment modalities and other pay-offs from stem cell research hold out significant
hope for the prevention, detection and treatment of disease. Furthermore, we
are aware of the revived threat of biological warfare and the new threats of
bioterrorism, as well as the new spectrum of worries related to deadly infectious diseases such as avian flu, mad cow disease, SARS, and Ebola. These
infectious threats create a need for new vaccines, new preventive measures,
and new treatments.

Those who consider the potential for advances in today's less than ideal
medical treatments, immunization, and disease prevention, recognize that almost everyone would want medicine to be able to provide effective treatment
when she or he or loved ones should need it. And from the recognition that
their compatriots are subject to the same biological vulnerabilities and that
they too would want medical interventions for themselves and their loved
ones, beneficence directs that the benefits that medicine can provide should be
made available to others in their society with medical needs. Yet, without human subject research, those treatments are far less likely to be available. So, in
light of the appreciation of human vulnerability to injury and disease and the

appreciation of the value of clinical research, every reasonable person should endorse policies that make research participation a social duty.[6]

In the same way that we have endorsed laws that require us to pay taxes and to serve on juries, people should accept an obligation to periodic service as research subjects. In an age when it is important to learn about the long-term effects of therapies and the unusual side-effects and complications that may not appear in the time-limited Phase-3 drug trials that try to identify them, and when population studies will be crucial for identifying the genetic component of disease and crucial for improving the efficacy of medical therapy through pharmaco-genetics, we need general cooperation in the project of advancing medical science.

To withhold endorsement from such a policy and to rely upon other means for human subject research that target the poor, the ill, the uninformed, and a few self-sacrificing altruists for serving as research subjects takes advantage of their vulnerability, gullibility and kindness. In that sense, the present voluntary participation system allows and even encourages people to behave as free-riders[7] by relying on others to bear the risks and burdens while those who are less civic-minded are free to share in the benefits produced by the research enterprise. The current practice, which relies exclusively on voluntary participation, allows research beneficiaries to ignore the moral equality of others by seeing those who participate as fodder and themselves as worthy beneficiaries of research subjects' sacrifice. In that we are biologically similar to each other, which makes the knowledge gained from studying others applicable to us, and that the biological differences between us, for the most part, have no moral significance, being a free-rider is unreasonable, and hence, immoral. In the sense that no rational person could withhold agreement to research participation without injustice, it is fair and just to institute a policy for reasonable research participation so that everyone is compelled to do a fair part.

Certainly, a policy of required service as a research subject would have to be significantly different from plans for paying taxes. Unlike money, our bodies are not fungible. Some physical requirements will be crucial for some projects (e.g., subjects might be restricted to women, those with glaucoma, or a serious burn). Yet, because almost everyone would want to share in the benefits of medical science, and because no one can be certain about the specific nature of her own or her loved ones' future medical needs, each should be expected to do her part in contributing to the advance of medical science that requires research with human subjects.

4. The Place of Informed Consent under a Decent Research Policy

Although my proposal would require everyone's participation in research, informed consent would still play an important role in that people would be choosing the studies for discharging their participation commitment rather than being conscripted into studies by others. The policy's allowance for individual decision making expresses our commitments to liberty and respect for autonomy. In this framework, informed consent would still be a crucial component for the ethical conduct of human subject research. Its role, however, would be markedly different from the place it has been given since the Nuremberg Code.[8] Rather than taking informed consent to be the necessary tool for protecting vulnerable subjects from Nazi-like researchers, in the model I suggest informed consent would have four new and distinct functions.

(1) Providing potential subjects with the information they should have for making a decision about participation in a study would help to assure the trust and trustworthiness of biomedical research. In an informed consent environment, people would not volunteer to serve as research subjects or endorse and comply with a policy of required research participation unless they could trust biomedical research as an institution and the individual researchers who conducted studies under its auspices. Without subjects having good reason to trust that they were not likely to be significantly harmed or to experience more burdens than they had been given to expect and that the studies would actually produce valuable information, the research enterprise could not go forward. Developing subject trust and assuring the trustworthiness of biomedical research practices is, therefore, essential for the practice of human subject research.

Medical science's need for trust and medical researchers' need for trust provides the reasons for assuring the trustworthiness of their practice.[9] For research to be trustworthy, medical science has to take its fiduciary responsibility seriously and pay significant attention to research oversight (e.g., by Institutional Review Boards, henceforth, IRBs). The scientific community's commitment to the trustworthy conduct of research allows subjects to be reasonably confident that the studies in which they enroll will impose no unreasonable risks or burdens, that each research project will be well designed, properly conducted, and could conceivably produce its promised results.[10]

(2) We know that the same thing can look very different from different perspectives. From the point of view of a researcher, whose judgment may be colored by self-interest or theoretical commitments,[11] or even a relatively objective review body, some risks and burdens could appear quite reasonable. Yet, they might appear not quite so reasonable from the point of view of some potential subjects. Allowing subjects the option of choosing their participation with full disclosure, of at least the usual kinds of information required by cur-

rent regulations and guidelines, would allow their judgment to serve as a check on researcher bias.[12]

(3) Informed and voluntary selection of projects by subject-participants would keep research design to an ethically reasonable standard because researchers would be reluctant to publicly describe procedures that they should not undertake. When subjects are kept in the dark and researchers can conceal the nature of what they are doing behind masks of deception and duplicity, some researchers could be tempted to do things they otherwise would not. In the light of full disclosure, a well-nurtured sense of shame is likely to inhibit those who might be tempted to stretch the moral limits. In this way, a publicity condition that makes research proposals transparent to the biomedical research community, to the public, and to the prospective subjects inhibits researchers from undertaking unreasonable studies.

(4) Informed consent would also be the principal mechanism for permitting people liberty and assuring respect for subject autonomy. It would allow individuals to fulfill their research obligations within a framework that recognizes and values the broad range of human goals and commitments. Family responsibilities, career agendas, personal projects, tastes, attitudes toward risk and pain, and an assortment of other individual concerns could make some particular project choices reasonable and acceptable to some and different ones reasonable and acceptable to others. For a person who has suffered from schizophrenia and found the burdens associated with current drug regimes very onerous, the risks associated with a drug-free wash out period for a trial of a new drug could be worth taking. For another with a family history of Alzheimer's disease, the discomfort and inconvenience of a study that could advance the scientific understanding of that particular degenerative process could be worth taking. For someone else, it could be important to find a project that could be done from home or completed within a single day. For another, a study that involved new technology (for instance, PET scans) would be most interesting. And for another, the more human interaction the better. Leaving the judgment to the involved individuals is likely to actually expand the parameters of acceptable research beyond those set by today's disinterested "protectors" of research subjects because individuals' personal values and personal attitudes toward risk vary significantly. That's precisely the point of valuing liberty and respecting autonomy.

5. The Autonomy Objections

I fully expect that there will be readers who view the ethical conduct of human subject research in terms of the currently accepted doctrines and, therefore, see my proposal as immoral. Some critics of my proposal for universal required participation in biomedical research may see it as a violation of autonomy, in that it would require participation even from those who would prefer not serving as a research subject. That stand would, however, miss the point of autonomy as the rule-giving, self-legislating capacity to undertake responsibility and to create influences to control one's own behavior. Every principle and every policy that a person endorses constrains her own future behavior. That's what every personal commitment does, and it is what all laws do. Most people do want biomedical science to pursue therapeutic advances, and they are prepared to do their fair share when others do so as well. So, when a person seriously considers the proposal as well as the alternatives, and then endorses a policy of required research participation, compliance and even compulsory participation do not violate autonomy because it is the rule that the person legislates for herself. Just as other laws compel compliance from those who previously endorsed them in one way or another, there is no obvious reason why a research participation policy should be different. Neither laws nor policies that one endorses violate autonomy by requiring compliance when the laws or policies are, in fact, the expression of an autonomous choice.

6. The Liberty Objection

> Oh duty,
> Why hast thou not the visage of a sweetie or a cutie?
> *Kind of an Ode to Duty,* Ogden Nash

In *On Liberty*, John Stuart Mill argues for the importance of liberty and that the prevention of harm to others is the only legitimate justification for a state's infringement on liberty.[13] Those, including Matti Häyry, who embrace Mill's view might join me in acknowledging the importance of research participation. Yet, I expect that Matti and those who share Mill's perspective would balk at the idea of making it mandatory and compelling participation. They could actually find an infringement on liberty for the sake of advancing the common good to be immoral. I also appreciate that many want to avoid hearing that they have to, or that they must, do anything. People often share Ogden Nash's sentiment and would rather accept the gentler conclusion that it would be nice if you would participate, or that you'd be a dear if you would sign on, but it's totally up to you.

Although I agree that safeguarding liberty is a very important ethical consideration, I also believe that doing some things is sometimes a matter of duty. There are also factors beyond harm to others that can sometimes justify overriding individual liberty.

In the case of research participation, at least three significant reasons justify limiting liberty: the importance of advancing biomedical science for the common good, the moral importance of equality with the concomitant problem of injustice created by free-riders, and the need for general cooperation for the success of the project. Whereas my presentation above inherently incorporated all three threads, allow me to tease them apart to further clarify the need for accepting research participation as a duty and the ground for a mandatory participation policy.

Advancing the Common Good. Because almost everyone and almost all of their loved ones has medical needs at some point in their lives, and because we frequently cannot know in advance which medical needs any particular subject will have in the future, and because researchers sometimes need to study subjects who are ill, sometimes subjects from different genetic groups, and sometimes entire populations, participation in research should be seen as a *prima facie* social duty. Medical needs are very widely appreciated. Sometimes a medical need is related to a genetic predisposition, sometimes some accident of life. Nevertheless, when a person perceives the need to have a condition of the body alleviated, they want the means to be available to address the problem, and today many conditions cannot be satisfactorily addressed with currently available interventions. Yet, advancing the good that medicine can do can only be achieved by studying our bodies. Whereas other social obligations can be fulfilled in other ways (e.g., by writing a check, by sending a stand-in, by paying for someone else's labor), at a certain point in biomedical research, there is nothing that we can substitute for us. Study involves some sacrifice of our flesh, our privacy, our safety, our comfort, and our time.

Because these basic goods that medicine can provide are precious to everyone, non-instrumental basic moral principles of equality, universalization, and mutual love require us to give of ourselves as we would wish to receive from others. For those reasons, every one should accept responsibility for doing her fair share so as to further the common good of biomedical science from which we expect ourselves and our loved ones to ultimately benefit. In sum, the fragility of our bodies, the invasiveness of research, our emotional and genetic interrelatedness, the lack of an adequate alternative, and the commonality of the desire to benefit from medical knowledge combine to create the participatory duty. Ethically speaking, when something is a duty, it is no longer optional, it is morally required.

The practice of medicine is advanced by research. When physicians and patients acknowledge and accept that treatment in the context of research offers our best hope for advancing the field we will be significantly more likely to improve medical knowledge. As an illustration, consider the field of organ transplantation. Given the severe shortage of cadaveric transplant organs together with the growing demand for transplantation and retransplantation, it becomes crucial to learn about conditions that are likely to promote graft and patient survival and factors that are likely to predict organ rejection and other problems. The model of research joined hand in hand with treatment that I am advocating would consider every organ recipient as a patient and also as a collaborator in the ongoing research effort. A treatment approach that also embraces research would allow clinician researchers to store and identify specimens and records for later use in projects that have not yet been conceived, to follow-up with identifiable previous organ recipients to help confirm or disconfirm hypotheses, and to re-contact patients when they are needed to help further future research goals. Because those who hope to benefit from receiving an organ transplant are beneficiaries of not only the donated transplant organ, but also the knowledge already gained from the study of previously transplanted patients, and because opportunities to advance this field should not be wasted, everyone who hopes to receive a transplant organ also has an obligation to participate in transplant research.

On this view the social purpose of biomedical research is a legitimate goal for medicine, and advancing that goal requires accepting a moral duty to do one's fair share. Saying that we each have an obligation to participate in biomedical research implies that clinicians should invite or even urge patients to participate in research and that patients who refuse to participate have to justify their refusal at least to themselves. Without going so far as actually adopting my proposal, this suggested change in attitude toward research puts the onus on the opposite side of where it has been under current conceptions of the ethics of research. Once the social purpose of research is accepted as a legitimate ground for a participatory duty, the next questions are who has such a duty, and what measures to assure compliance are justified?

Equality. Although people are all different from each other in many ways, they are similar enough to one another to be considered as if they were equal in two important respects. First, biologically, people are all mortal, they are all vulnerable to death, disease, and injury, and they all can experience pain, suffering, and disability. Furthermore, the function of organs and the biophysiological processes in one human is very much like the function and processes in another. These biological factors make us roughly fungible equivalents for purposes of medical treatment and biomedical research. What is learned on one of us can be used later to benefit another.

Second, ethically, for the most part, at least among those who are capable of abiding by moral rules and actually treating others as they think they should, the differences between us are not significant enough to amount to a moral difference in how we should treat one another: Every one is owed caring and respect from others. Given these two sources of equality, we are morally bound to treat one another as we would have others treat us. This is the basic standard of morality.

Since we each would want medicine to be advanced enough to respond effectively to whatever medical needs we should develop, and since treatment advances necessarily involve human subject research, given our biological and moral equality, we should not expect others to contribute their bodies when we are not willing to do so as well. Accepting the medical advances of research on others, when one has not contributed her own body in reasonably safe studies, would be taking advantage of their participation without doing one's fair share, benefiting from the contributions of others while not contributing in kind. That is the essence of being a free-rider, it amounts to treating others unjustly by denying their moral equality. Hence, we are each required to do unto others as we would have others do unto us, which, in this case means that we each have a duty to participate in biomedical research, at least when the oversight is adequate and when the studies are reasonably safe.

Collaborative Necessity. There are many projects that can be accomplished alone or in concert with just a few other individuals. Bench research and animal studies surely fall into that category. Paying a salary is sufficient to accomplish some of the tasks that require the participation of others. Many Phase-1 drug studies could be conducted with paid subjects.[14] But other kinds of research require people who actually have one condition or another. And in some circumstances the risks and burdens of a study can only be justified when it is performed on those whose serious or deteriorating medical condition leaves them in a situation with little to lose, or perhaps lots to gain, from exposure to the risks involved in a study. And in many situations, such as when researchers are trying to determine unusual side effects of a drug, or subtle differences in responses of alternative treatments, or the effects of some environmental change on an entire population, or learn about the effectiveness of treatment for some relatively rare condition, it is clear that everyone, or everyone in the target group should participate as study subjects.

The achievement of numerous societal goods requires general cooperation. Sometimes general cooperation is intrinsic to the good that is to be achieved. For example, everyone must obey the criminal law in order to create the safety and stability that the criminal law protects. Sometimes the justification is structural. For example, to assure that every one accused of a crime can be tried by peers, no individuals or groups can be privileged to opt out of jury service. Sometimes general cooperation is required merely for reasons of efficacy. For example, it would be too costly to provide non-fluoridated water to those who want to avoid the chemical. Sometimes the requirement for doing one's fair share is justified by the great good that cannot be achieved without general cooperation. Roads, schools, environmental protection, sanitation services, a standing army, emergency management services, centers for disease control, boards of elections, and an array of other services supported by taxes are all instances of social goods that require funding from the general public. Other social benefits require general behavioral compliance: observing traffic regulations, abstaining from littering, cleaning up after your dog. Sometimes a social good cannot be achieved when some are allowed to opt out. Water and air pollution may be threatened by the exemption of even a few individuals.

In all such cases, the need for general cooperation justifies limitations on individual liberty, even though harm to others would only apply as a justification in a few examples. Because of the significant and important social good that can be achieved through general cooperation in biomedical research, and because important opportunities for advancing biomedical science are likely to be squandered without widespread participation, requiring participation is well justified.

Furthermore, given that humans are all also susceptible to seeing the burdens on themselves as very significant while minimizing the burdens endured by others, and given the human tendency to avoid duty and to justify their avoidance with a variety of creative excuses, it is easy to appreciate the need for establishing coercive mechanisms to get ourselves to do just what we think we should do. In the philosophic literature, such constraints are commonly described as Ulysses contracts for their similarity to the way Ulysses arranged to have himself fettered so that he would be prevented from doing what he thought he should not do. For Ulysses, having himself bound to the mast was his autonomous choice. Nevertheless, when he wanted to be at liberty to follow the Sirens' song, he was restrained from doing what he chose at the moment. Any rules that we endorse for constraining our own future actions can be seen as Ulysses contracts. In the limited sense of interference with a present choice, such rules do impede liberty. But in a more generous and far-sighted sense, the rules that we endorse after our own considered reflection should be seen as the expressions of our liberty even when they restrict our behavior at a moment when we would prefer to be free of our bonds.

Required research participation could be just such an instance, and, perhaps for this conjunction of reasons, even Häyry could freely endorse a policy of required research participation.

7. Concern for Vulnerable Subjects

Some who reject my proposal may have reservations of an entirely different sort and see it as immoral because it would require participation from everyone. In line with the current standards that appear to have been formulated primarily to avoid the abuse of Nazi doctors who used concentration camp inmates as test subjects, such critics take the proper aim of research standards to be the protection of vulnerable subjects from being abused by unscrupulous researchers. Such objectors are likely to hold that some individuals should not be subjects in biomedical research, or enrolled in only the most benign projects, because of their vulnerability. The crux of this objection is that the vulnerable are entitled to special protections, whereas my decent proposal for the conduct of human subject research in a just society urges broad inclusion across the population.

The reigning view expressed in current human subject research regulations is that regulatory attention should focus on protecting the vulnerable. However, this has also been identified as an antiliberal Marxist element in research ethics.[15] Even the titles of oversight policies and agencies reflect this narrow aim. In the U.S., the regulations are called "Policy for the Protection of

Human Research Subjects,"[16] and the agency for compliance was first the Office for the Protection from Research Risks (OPRR) and now the Office for Human Research Protection (OHRP). Although there is an obvious intuitive appeal in the desire to protect those who are least able to protect themselves, current research policies too often limit research, particularly with individuals who are classified as "vulnerable," and thereby promote practices that are unethical and unreasonable by being harmful, wasteful, or both. Rather than according a reasonable balance to a range of interrelated issues that affect the moral assessment of various projects, (e.g., risk, efficacy, justice, respect), the rules give special weight to the protection of the vulnerable.

Under the banner of informed consent, the U.S. Department of Health and Human Services has increasingly moved its regulatory attention in the direction of protecting human research subjects from coercive pressures or harms. Parents should certainly protect their children. But, consider the bike riding policy that parents would adopt if they took protection to be their primary parental responsibility. Children would not be allowed to ride bikes because it would subject them to risk of harm. Parents who actually allow their children to ride are likely to consider the importance of protection and also the importance of other developmental goals such as: independence, risk management, social interaction, and exploration. When a multiplicity of goals is accepted, protection is considered in the context of other critical objectives and other aims will sometimes be overriding, particularly when potential subjects who are perceived as vulnerable.[17]

Presumably, certain groups cannot be expected to understand or appreciate information about proposed research projects, and that makes them vulnerable to exploitation and abuse. OPRR, and the newly created OHRP have reaffirmed protectionist commitments. According to their policies, and those of IRBs that introduce additional policies inspired by the regulations, vulnerable groups include: the mentally ill, the mentally handicapped, pregnant women, fetuses, products of in vitro fertilization, children, prisoners, the elderly, people who are in the midst of a medical emergency, and the educationally or economically disadvantaged. That's a lot of people. Even more vigorous efforts to protect vulnerable subjects of research are urged by non-governmental groups such as the Alliance for Human Research Protection.

Although the regulations express legitimate concerns about the potential for harm, force, and deception, the efforts to protect the vulnerable are guided by a distorted view of the significance of informed consent. Some groups that are classified as "vulnerable" clearly lack decisional capacity. For that reason, research involving children, the profoundly retarded, the seriously mentally ill, the demented, and the unconscious clearly need special oversight. But protecting research subjects from other groups based on their classification as "vulnerable" does not show respect for their autonomy and concern for liberty. It is actually a denigration of their autonomy and an infringement on their liberty.

Protective policy presumes that the vulnerable are unable to appreciate and assess risks and that judgment of benefits and burdens should, therefore, be made by others. This is paternalism. It denies people the opportunity to evaluate the costs and benefits of research participation in light of their own priorities, their own goals, and their own values. Instead of respecting the autonomy of others by assuming that they are autonomous, classifying people as "vulnerable" denies them the ethically required default presumption, that they can make decisions that reflect their own values and commitments.

The outlandishness of this approach to groups designated as "vulnerable" becomes vivid when we notice that pregnant women are presumed to have the capacity to make choices about child bearing, that the mentally ill are frequently allowed to make choices about their living arrangements, and that restrictions on the liberty of the elderly or the educationally or economically disadvantaged in any circumstances other than consent to research would be branded unacceptable discrimination. Although some who can be included in these groups may lack decisional capacity, evaluation cannot be based on group membership. The determination must be predicated on a demonstration that the particular individual in question is not entitled to be presumed autonomous or, for some reason, lacks the capacity to make a decision about research participation in particular.[18]

Respect for another as an autonomous being requires allowing that person to make choices about research participation policy by assessing the personal and societal disadvantages and advantages involved. This permits individuals to factor their personal values and experience into their choice. When those engaged in research oversight in the name of autonomy take the stance of "protector," they express a willingness to deny genuine respect for autonomy out of fear of possibly allowing someone to make a less than ideally autonomous choice. However, as Mill and Häyry have taught us, respect for liberty requires the opposite approach by recognizing the illegitimacy of limitations on personal choice out of concern for the personal safety of others.

Yet, today's research subject "protectors" seek ever more demanding mechanisms of protection and search out more and more groups that may be less than ideally rational and, so, in need of their protection. These well-meaning efforts are misdirected and counter-productive in that many may do more harm than good by curtailing liberty and disrespecting autonomous choices. This fact is demonstrated in the U.S. by many people who suffer from one disease or another organizing disease-based groups (e.g., the mentally ill) to advocate for more research on their condition and fewer restrictions on participation.

I am suggesting instead that regulative attention be directed at the development of reasonable boundaries for the conduct of human subject research. Rather than focusing narrowly on the protection of vulnerable subjects, IRBs should prohibit everyone from participation in studies that are unreasonably risky or burdensome. So long as this gate-keeper function is seriously addressed, every approved study should involve only acceptable risks so that no subjects are exposed to excessive risks. For the most part, if it would be acceptable for someone who has decisional capacity to participate in a study, it should also be reasonable for a surrogate to enroll a subject who lacks decisional capacity. If the risks and burdens make it unacceptable for someone who has decisional capacity to participate in a study, it should also be unacceptable for a surrogate to enroll a subject who lacks decisional capacity. As a general rule, if it would be acceptable for a capacitated patient to choose, or for a surrogate to authorize or forgo an innovative therapeutic intervention, then it should also be reasonable to enroll a subject who lacks decisional capacity in a trial of that therapy when research involves only reasonably small additional burdens. Beyond these limitations, while largely allowing decisions to reside with surrogates, research policy should elaborate on additional oversight precisely because subjects who lack decisional capacity are unable to judge for themselves when the risks and burdens of an ongoing study are or become unreasonable.

Prisoners are a special case. On the one hand, prisoners with a particular disease condition (e.g., HIV) may very much want to participate in a study of a new intervention. On the other hand, because every aspect of their lives is controlled by others, it is hard to see how they could provide genuine consent. Also, the importance of keeping the criminal justice system free of contaminating influences, could justify restricting the participation of prisons in clinical research.

Lack of autonomy is an excellent reason for refusing to leave decisions about research participation with those who lack decisional capacity. It does not, however, justify a limitation on their research participation. IRBs should examine protocols with an eye toward prohibiting those studies that would impose an unreasonable risk and significant harm and devote attention to oversight of ongoing studies. When IRBs actually embraced these responsibilities, they would permit only research with reasonable risks and burdens to go forward. This new approach would leave neither the decisionally competent nor the decisionally incompetent without protection: Everyone would be protected from unreasonable risks and burdens. Regulations and IRB review and oversight would protect all individuals from unreasonable harms. This paternalistic protection would not be justified by protecting those who lack decisional capacity (i.e., what has been called "soft paternalism") but by the significant social benefit achieved by preserving the trustworthiness of biomedical science. In other words, this is an imposition on those who should be presumed to be autonomous, hence, "hard paternalism." In such an environment, the worry about accepting the consent of someone who was less than ideally autonomous would be negligible because protections against exposure to unreasonable risk would be in place.

Parents who allow their children to ride bikes, may impose limitations that reflect a concern about protection from excessive or likely risks. Parents may restrict bike riding to bike paths and require children to wear helmets. Similarly, IRBs can impose limits on research or prohibit studies that expose subjects to excessive or likely significant risks. The changes in IRB responsibility that I am suggesting would involve additional expertise, training, staffing, and monitoring to provide the appropriate level of review and oversight. The details of how these costs can be met goes beyond the scope of this discussion.

8. Objections to the Enrollment of Children in Research

Reigning policies restrict the participation of children in biomedical research because children are vulnerable. By definition, children are not (fully) autonomous, so they cannot consent to research themselves.

The most obvious consequence of these rules is that pediatricians are frequently left to treat children with no data to support the choice of treatment or dosage of prescribed medications. Treatment protocols and dose rates of medications are typically developed in studies of adult men. But children are significantly different from adult men, and a modification in treatment or reduction in dosage to reflect only the difference in weight may ignore other significant differences between children and adults. Adult bodies are fully developed, but the bodies of children are developing in ways that could be impacted differently by a treatment or drug depending upon their particular stage of development. Children are, typically, a lot more active than adult men. Their metabolism is different, their diet may be different. Because they are young, children can be expected to live with treatment and drug effects longer than adults will, and the long-term toxicity could be significantly different from a shorter effect.

Without information about the effect of an intervention on each of these variables, pediatricians are left to develop their idiosyncratic accumulation of guesses and anecdotes. Pediatricians are unable to extrapolate from studies on capacitated similar subjects because there are none. This perpetuation of the *status quo* leaves each treated child to face otherwise avoidable dangers. It is hard to see how continually subjecting children to the risks of shooting in the dark can be a more ethical approach than developing evidence to guide clinical pediatric practice through research involving children.

9. Conclusions

To the extent that my arguments in support of the decent proposal for the conduct of human subject research are persuasive, and to the extent that my responses to the expected objections of those who would find it immoral are compelling, the proposal should be endorsed. With an appreciation of both the dangers and the promises of research we can advance our understanding of the ethical conduct of human subject research and, thereby, advance our knowledge of biomedical science. This new framework will require us to see researchers and subjects as cooperative partners engaged in and committed to socially important collaborative projects constrained within bounds of reasonable risk.[19] It will also require IRBs to appreciate their charge as protectors of the trust and trustworthiness of the biomedical research enterprise. This new role will require increased attention to the evaluation of the scientific merits and conduct of studies, the assessment of potential risks and burdens, and investment into oversight of ongoing projects.

At this point in our evolving understanding of the moral requirements for the ethical conduct of human subject research it is crucial that we carefully assess the claims about immorality that have become the regulatory ideology. At the same time, it is crucial that we rethink the requirements for the ethical conduct of research with sensitivity to complexity and awareness of the range of contexts in which clinical studies are and should be conducted. At the very least, my proposal should press us to reexamine and reassess the reigning research dogmas. In the face arguments I have offered, cleaving to the old web of dogmas as the justification for policy cannot be justified.

Human subject research remains an inherently risky business which also makes rethinking research ethics risky. One hazard comes from the powerful amalgamated political and economic interests in biomedical research which have succeeded in limiting the applicability of the current U.S. standards to the signatory agencies (e.g., it still has not been fully accepted by the Environmental Protection Agency) and preventing the Common Rule from becoming a national standard (e.g., it does not apply to research done entirely with privately funding). These forces can be expected to try to control, distort and subvert reform efforts.

Another hazard comes from the difficulty of grasping the complexity of what is involved in research ethics and the opposing inclination to seize onto clear, simple, or popular definitions and solutions. In any effort to rethink and improve upon our current system, it is also very easy to overlook important considerations or to fail to foresee all of the consequences of a well-intentioned change.

As Matti Häyry has repeatedly demonstrated, ethics is not simple. People easily latch onto poorly understood vague concepts and use them carelessly without adequately appreciating their implications. The desire to do good can be perverted and distorted. Thoughtful analysis and careful consideration of the meaning of our terms, the reasonableness of our beliefs, and the implications of our policies are our only defense against our vulnerability to committing the serious errors in moral reasoning. When we do ultimately recognize our errors, courageous and timely correction is in order.

ACKNOWLEDGEMENT

Preliminary work on this paper was presented as, "Rethinking Informed Consent for Research," first at the International Bioethics Retreat, Florence, Italy, October 4, 1999, and a later, fuller version that was read at Davidson College, November 5, 1999. A far more complex critique of current research regulation appeared as "Rethinking Research Ethics" in *American Journal of Bioethics*. I thank Matti Häyry, Joe Fitschen, Ian Holzman, and Jonathan Rhodes, as well as the members of those audiences, for their comments and suggestions.

NOTES

1. Matti Häyry, "A Rational Cure for Pre-Reproductive Stress Syndrome," *Journal of Medical Ethics*, 30 (2004), pp. 377–378.

2. Rosamond Rhodes, "Rethinking Research Ethics" (Target Article), *American Journal of Bioethics*, 5:1 (2005), pp. 7–28.

3. Matti Häyry, *Liberal Utilitarianism and Applied Ethics* (London: Routledge, 1994).

4. Tuija Takala and Matti Häyry, "Genetic Ignorance, Moral Obligations and Social Duties," *Journal of Medicine and Philosophy*, 25 (2000), pp. 107–113.

5. Matti Häyry, "Abortion, Disability, Assent and Consent," *Cambridge Quarterly of Healthcare Ethics*, 10 (2001): 79–87.

6. See Arthur Caplan, "Is There a Duty to Serve as a Subject in Biomedical Research?" *IRB: Ethics and Human Research*, 6:5 (1984), pp. 1–5.

7. Paul Menzel, "Justice and the Basic Structure of Health-Care Systems," *Medicine and Social Justice: Essays on the Distribution of Health Care*, eds. R. Rhodes, M. P. Battin, and A. Silvers (New York: Oxford University Press, 2002), pp. 24–37.

8. See, *e.g.* George J. Annas, Leonard H. Glantz, Barbara Katz, *Informed Consent to Human Experimentation: The Subject's Dilemma* (Cambridge, MA: Ballinger Publishing company, 1977); Paul Appelbaum, Charles Lidz, and Alan Meisel, *Informed Consent: Legal Theory and Clinical Practice* (New York: Oxford University Press, 1987); Baruch A. Brody, *The Ethics of Biomedical Research: An International Perspective* (New York: Oxford University Press, 1998); Ruth R. Faden and Tom L. Beauchamp, *A History and Theory of Informed Consent* (New York: Oxford University Press, 1986); Albert R. Jonsen, *The Birth of Bioethics* (New York: Oxford University Press 1998); Albert R. Jonsen, "The Ethics of Research with Human Subjects: A Short History," *Source Book in Bioethics: A Documentary History*, eds. Albert R. Jonsen, Robert M. Veatch, and LeRoy Walters (Washington, DC: Georgetown University Press, 1998), pp. 5–10; David J. Rothman, *Strangers at the Bedside* (New York: Basic Books, 1991); Ulf I. Schmidt, *Justice at Nuremberg: Leo Alexander and the Nazi Doctors' Trial* (Palgrave/Macmillan, forthcoming); Adil E. Shamoo and David B. Resnik, "The Use of Human Subjects in Research," *Responsible Conduct of Research*. (New York: Oxford, 2003), pp. 181–208; Robert Veatch, *The Patient as Partner: A Theory of Human-Experimentation Ethics* (Bloomington: Indian University Press, 1987); and

Hans Jonas, "Philosophical Reflections on Experimenting with Human Subjects," *Deadalus: Journal of the American Academy of Arts and Sciences*, Spring 1969, pp. 219–247, cited from Ronald Munson, *Intervention and Reflection: Basic Issues in Medical Ethics*, sixth edition (Belmont: Wadsworth, 2000), pp. 499–508.

9. Stephan Fuchs and Saundra Davis Westervelt, "Fraud and Trust in Science," *Perspectives in Biology and Medicine*, 39 (1996), pp. 248–269; Rosamond Rhodes and James Strain, "Trust and Transforming Medical Institutions," *Cambridge Quarterly of Healthcare Ethics*, 9 (2000), pp. 205–217.

10. Benjamin Freedman, Abraham Fuks, and Charles Weijer, "In Loco Parentis: Minimal Risk as an Ethical Threshold for Research upon Children," *Hastings Center Report*, 23 (1993), pp. 13–19; p. 18.

11. Peter Brian Medawar, "Scientific Fraud," in his *The Threat and the Glory* (New York: Harper Collins, 1983), pp. 64–70; p. 65.

12. See also Jay Katz, "Abuse of Human Beings for the Sake of Science," *When Medicine Went Mad*, ed. Arthur L. Caplan (Totowa: Humana Press, 1992), pp. 233–270; p. 257.

13. John Stuart Mill, *On Liberty*, ed. Elizabeth Rapaport (Indianapolis: Hackett Publishing Company, 1978).

14. Trudo Lemmens, "Justice for the Professional Guinea Pig," *The American Journal of Bioethics*, 1 (2001), pp. 51–53; Trudo Lemmens and Carl Elliott, "Guinea Pigs on the Payroll: The Ethics of Paying Research Subjects," *Accountability in Research*, 7 (1991), pp. 3–20; Ruth Macklin, "On Paying Money to Research Subjects: 'Due' and 'Undue' Inducements," *IRB: Ethics and Human Research*, 3 (May 1981), pp. 1–6; Julian Savulescu, "The Fiction of 'Undue Inducement': Why Researchers Should Be Allowed to Pay Participants Any Amount of Money for Any Reasonable Research Project," *The American Journal of Bioethics*, 1 (2001): on line.

15. Madison Powers, *Beyond Consent: Seeking Justice in Research* (New York: Oxford University Press, 1997), pp. 151–152.

16. U.S. Department of Health and Human Services, Code of Federal Regulations, Title 45, Public Welfare Act, Part 46, Protection of Human Subjects (Common Rule), Revised June 23, 2005.

17. *Cf.* Robert J. Levine, "Adolescents as Research Subjects without Permission of Their Parents or Guardians: Ethical Considerations," *Journal of Adolescent Health*, 17 (1995), pp. 287–297; Robert J. Levine, "Some Recent Developments in the International Guidelines on the Ethics of Research Involving Human Subjects," *Annals of the New York Academy of Science*, 918 (2000), pp. 170–178.

18. See, Dave Wendler and Kiran Prasad, "Core Safeguards for Clinical Research with Adults Who Are Unable To Consent," *Annals of Internal Medicine*, 135 (2001), pp. 514–523.

19. See also Katz, "Abuse of Human Beings for the Sake of Science," p. 258.

Part Five

RATIONALITY, MORALITY,
AND REPRODUCTION

Sixteen

PARENTAL RESPONSIBILITY AND THE DUTY TO LOVE ONE'S CHILDREN

Floora Ruokonen and Simo Vehmas

1. Introduction

Not all children are accepted as they are by their parents. Although the ideal of an unqualified, whole-hearted parental love is probably widely accepted in the Western world, very few of us who have children can claim to consistently fulfill this ideal in practice. Various qualities in our children may annoy us; some of us wish to have children of a certain sex or with certain aptitudes, such as talent for music or math. In these kinds of cases, having a child with a "wrong" sex or "wrong" kind of aptitudes may be difficult to accept. Some may even have difficulties of cultivating loving emotions toward their child whom they find ugly or resembling someone they loathe.

Nowadays the highly advanced medicine can, to some extent, help parents to fulfill their wishes regarding the qualities of their potential children. In practice this means that prenatal diagnosis can provide parents with information concerning the characteristics of their potential child, and on the basis of this information, they may choose to terminate the pregnancy (i.e., selective abortion). Prenatal diagnosis has probably in its part increased the mixed emotions of many parents toward procreation and parenting; on the other hand they may think that they should be willing to accept any kind of child they will get, and be capable of loving him or her unconditionally. But then, if the parents can avoid, with the help of medicine, the birth of a child with undesirable characteristics, would not they be foolish *not* to seize the opportunity?

Ideas of parental duties, responsibilities and virtues have entered bioethical discussions in connection with new reproductive technologies, especially when the aim is to prevent the birth of children with certain characteristics. Apparently, there are two (possibly conflicting) discourses regarding parenthood and procreative autonomy. The official discourse among health care professionals emphasizes parental autonomy, self-determination and respect for privacy. Accordingly, people have the inalienable right to choose within certain time limits, for example, what kind of children they are willing to bear. On the other hand, in the Western culture parenthood is often seen to include the kind of virtues and duties that limit parents' choices; parents should commit themselves to parenting in the way that children's good comes always first. This could be seen to imply that potential parents should be willing to commit themselves to bearing and rearing children despite their characteristics.

Various philosophical arguments have been developed to support both of the discourses mentioned above. Rosamond Rhodes,[1] for example, has argued that a fetus's right to life is based on the mother's or both parents' assent to carry the pregnancy to term. According to this kind of assentist account, after assenting to the continuation of a pregnancy, the parents have accepted the responsibility to care for their offspring until it can be independent and able to assume obligations as a moral agent. The commitment to caring for and nurturing a child is (during the early pregnancy) conditional for parents: the assent given by the parents to care for a child applies only to the kind of child that will be able to become a moral agent. A child incapable of developing into a moral agent and living an independent life will become a lifelong burden to her parents. Imposing this kind of obligation on parents is, according to Rhodes, unreasonable. This being the case, the parents are morally justified in withdrawing the fetus's conditional right to life and withdrawing themselves from the parental position on the grounds of the fetus's impairment. They can, of course, make "a new act" by committing themselves to caring for a child who cannot become an independent moral agent. However, this kind of a renewed commitment seems to be in Rhodes's view more or less a supererogatory act.

Simo Vehmas has criticized Rhodes for being too permissive.[2] Vehmas argues that a conscious decision to procreate is an act of assent to commit oneself to the project of parenthood that includes certain responsibilities and obligations. Also, true parental assent cannot be conditional in the sense that people could commit themselves to parenting only a child of a certain kind, with pre-defined qualities and aptitudes. This implies that parents ought to commit themselves to caring unconditionally for any kind of child. Prospective parents who have decided to procreate are morally parents and they should have an unconditional attitude towards their prospective children in the same way as parents should take towards their actual children. According to Vehmas, this implies that selective abortion is *prima facie* morally wrong.

If one approaches the issue from a purely descriptive viewpoint, it is clear that a lot of people do not consider parenthood as an unconditional position or project. To many, impairment or gender is a proper reason to terminate pregnancy. These potential parents obviously do not think that they should accept or love unconditionally their future child despite of its characteristics. The general question directing the discussion in this paper is whether such parents are right or wrong. More specifically, our interest is the content of parental commitment and responsibility. We ask whether unconditional *love* for one's children is part of parental commitment and if it is, can it be posited as a parental duty? Finally we review a few possible implications that a positive answer to the above questions would have for the discussion concerning the moral justification of selective abortion.

2. Kant, Parenthood, and Pathological Love

To set a frame for the subsequent discussion, we will first briefly review assentism as a form of a Kantian theory. In both Rhodes' and Vehmas' accounts parental assent creates an obligation or a law to the parents for governing their action.[3] "The law" referred to here is a moral prescription, a duty, that a parent would accept when relying on her own pure reasoning. This means reasoning purified of self-seeking interests that might make it unjust or prejudiced. Clearly this is a Kantian model of arriving at moral judgments. The reasoning of an autonomous person (in the Kantian sense of the term) is the grounding of moral right and wrong. The issue, when it comes to the subject of this paper then is, as Matti Häyry has noted in his discussion of Rhodes' and Vehmas' positions, what exactly would the (ideally) reasonable person agree to were she to assents to the project of parenthood.[4] Good parenting is commonly thought to require love for one's children. But to answer the question of whether a rational person assenting to parenthood would also agree to love one's children, one would first have to answer the question whether it is possible to posit love as a duty. Since the assentist position is Kantian in its nature, it seems sensible to approach this question in the light of Kant's account of love.

The usual criticism levelled at Kant's moral theory is that it leaves very little room for emotions. However, various scholars have demonstrated that Kant actually assigned several important roles in his moral theory to emotions.[5] Kant did, nevertheless, see (particularly in *The Groundwork*) a particular group of emotions, which he referred to as inclinations, mostly as a nuisance which any rational being should avoid.[6] Inclinations are "habitual sensible desires"[7]; they are habitual, since the desire is associated with some object or state of affairs that the agent seeks to bring about because of some antecedent pleasures associated with it. They are sensible or "empirical" desires because they exist independently of reasoning or reflection.[8] Thus, they are not a matter of reason and active free will but, rather, the products of the passive and deterministic part of human beings. Inclinations have no role in the estimation of the moral worth of an agent, or his or her actions. In Kant's theory, moral worth is attributed to agents solely on the basis of being motivated by respect for duty. Human dignity is grounded on the autonomy of practical reason which is a faculty that enables human beings to legislate moral law for themselves. Respect for duty is the same as the recognition of the dignity of autonomous personhood in oneself, and in others.

So, from a Kantian perspective, morally worthy parenthood would be reduced to acting according to one's duty—and whatever the content of this duty is, love as an inclination would not be a part of it. However, a strict

Kantian view of the moral essence of parenthood causes at least two problems for a strong formulation of parental duties. First, neither fetuses nor newborn infants are persons in the Kantian sense. This being the case, they do not belong to the moral realm, they cannot be respected and one cannot have moral obligations towards them. Although this, in a sense, seems indisputable, it also leads to uncomfortable conclusions. If a pregnant mother has no obligations whatsoever to the fetus she carries, she would have no moral reason to restrain from using excessive amounts of drugs or any other habits that may harm the fetus. But it does seem that the mother has some sort of an obligation to consider her future child's well-being if she has decided to carry the pregnancy to term. Secondly, duties of respect towards persons are in Kant's theory *negative duties*, which are supposed to limit our actions; particularly they oblige us from injuring the dignity of other persons. However, this standpoint does not oblige persons, in this case the parents, to actively further other persons' (i.e. their child's) interests. But this seems counter-intuitive; surely parents are required to *actively* further their child's well-being. It also seems that if they intend to do this well, they should *love* their child. But does love have any place in Kant's moral theory and if it has, what does love mean within this theory?

Kant differentiates between two kinds of love, pathological and practical. *Pathological love* is an inclination, a feeling of pleasure or delight in the perfection of another and a disposition to benefit her on the basis of this pleasure. It is, in other words, a passive feeling. Since pathological love is "a matter of feeling, not of willing, and I cannot love because I will to, still less because I ought to (I cannot be constrained to love)," pathological love cannot be anybody's duty. So, as for pathological love, "a duty to love is an absurdity."[9] *Practical love*, however, can be a duty. Practical love refers to a desire to benefit another out of duty to act according to the maxim of benevolence.[10] When the moral agent "loves practically," she adopts the ends of another moral agent as her own; she recognizes a duty to further the good and the ends of another moral agent.

In sum, according to Kant we cannot (at least totally) control how and what we feel. Therefore, we cannot be obligated to have certain feelings. But since human beings are autonomous moral agents, they can be, and indeed are, obligated to act according to certain duties, of which practical love is one. Love in a moral sense, then, is not about feeling in a certain way but about acting in a certain way.[11]

Kant's account of love raises some concerns as for the moral essence of parenthood. Regardless of how love is defined, it seems intuitively clear that a genuine love for one's children should be an essential part of being a parent. This intuition can be supported with the following considerations: (1) The security that parental love brings allows children to flourish and to trust. (2) Parental love protects children, during childhood, from loneliness and isolation. (3) Whether or not parents love their children affects children's ability later to form and to maintain intimate relationships with others. (4) Parental love fosters children's developing self-respect.[12] Now, if it is true that parental love is needed for children to obtain the kind of benefits pointed above, and if there is a moral demand for parents to care to their best ability for the good of their children who are utterly dependent on them, love is one crucial requirement of parenting a child. And if this is the case, love ought to be a part of a moral theory concerning parenthood.

3. Is There a Duty to Cultivate Loving Emotions?

If one leans on Kant's theory, parents are obliged to act in a way which brings about the benefits mentioned above. The crucial moral issue is how they act toward their children, not what kinds of feelings they have for them. Now, it is logically possible that parents could act toward their child as if they felt love for her although, in fact, they do not. However this most probably would not work in practice because people (including children) usually can tell whether those near to them truly feel love for them or merely act as if they did. And to recognize that one's parents act out of duty in the way good parents should act, but actually do not have any "emotional warmth toward and connectedness with the child, genuine delight in the child herself,"[13] would probably be devastating to any child. It is very difficult to feign the feeling of love. Without heartfelt parental love children probably cannot *feel loved* by their parents. Since parental love is valuable to children, parents should actually feel love for their children.[14] In other words, parenthood seems to require, in Kantian terms, pathological love, tender sympathy as an inclination. Such love cannot, however, be posited as a duty.

At this point, it should be pointed out what we mean by emotions. Emotions have often been identified with feelings; they are visceral sensations that people are often able to feel in their bodies. For example, we *feel* jealous or angry; we can identify our emotional state by recognizing its physical symptoms (tightness in the stomach, rapid heart beat and so on). However, most emotions are differentiated by our beliefs and evaluations, not by how we feel. Our beliefs of what is, for instance, socially or morally appropriate, has a pivotal effect on our emotions. Because of this, we can often predict our feelings associated with certain actions. In other words, most of us would infer that if someone is caught stealing an acquaintance's wallet, she would feel shame. Thus, emotions are not just feelings, they include a cognitive component and thus rational component as well.[15]

Although Kant thinks that feelings cannot be willed and that therefore there cannot be a duty to have certain feelings, he does not think that they are totally beyond a person's own control. Kant suggests (in *The Metaphysics of Morals*) that moral agents have a duty to cultivate inclinations that enable them to more fittingly follow the duty dictated by reason.[16] Feelings or affections can be of help in motivating a person with the pursuit of fulfilling his or her duty of practical love. In this sense, feelings can be seen as useful in the Kantian framework, although they add nothing to the moral worth of fulfilling the duty.

We are ready to accept that there is no duty to love but, at the same time, we think that it is quite plausible to argue that people in certain positions have a duty to *try* to cultivate certain emotions, and accordingly feelings, that are in line with the demands of practical love. It is clear that people can, at least to some extent, cultivate and control their emotions. Because of this, they are also partly responsible for them. Cultivating one's emotions is possible because of the cognitive dimension related to them. By changing one's evaluations of a certain thing or person, one can often change one's emotions about it as well. This is not always easy, though. We are accustomed to react emotionally on the basis of our personal histories. Emotions are thus habits, in a way, and habits are not under our direct control. Habits are often deeply entrenched dispositions so learning to control and cultivate them can be very tricky, but not necessarily impossible.[17] However, since not all the factors affecting our emotions are under our control, responsibility for the *success* of the effort to cultivate one's emotions cannot be posited.

LaFollette defines love as "a disposition to act lovingly, a disposition which typically causes, or is associated with, loving feelings."[18] If it is assumed (like we assume) that love is a crucial disposition in a parental role and if it is assumed that one can to some extent cultivate such a disposition and the concomitant feelings, how is one to do that in practice? A rough answer could go as what follows. We must learn to understand why we feel as we do in certain situations and with respect to certain people. Without an understanding of one's emotional processes, one does not have control over them. So, when we know what and why we feel, we have the chance of altering the way we feel. After that, "we can deliberately develop emotional capacities through choosing to undertake activities typically associated with the capacities we want to engender."[19] Now, if a potential parent feels that she would not be capable of loving a child with, say, Down syndrome, she could attempt to do the following: First, the parent should try to understand why she actually finds it more difficult to love a child with Down syndrome than without it. What does she know about Down syndrome? Is her lore of Down syndrome based on appropriate knowledge or on mere stereotypes? Has she ever spent time with a child with Down syndrome? Would her emotions and feelings about parenting a child with a Down syndrome change if she actually spent time with such children, considered them as unique individuals with interests and rights of their own, and acted accordingly? Finally, she might want to ask what the idea of good parenthood means to her: is it something conditional, something that depends on the "normality" of the child?

We do not intend to suggest that successful cultivation of loving emotions and feelings is a duty. Nevertheless, since parental love is of crucial importance in being a parent, perhaps one could require that parents should at least *try* to cultivate loving emotions and feelings toward their child, irrespective of their (actual or potential) child's characteristics.

Emotions are not only a part of the project of parenthood; they also structure and inform our conceptions of the project itself. Making parental and procreative choices is not a matter of mere rationality—emotions and feelings play a noteworthy part in it. In order to address properly questions related to procreation, such as the question of the justification of selective abortion, one should acknowledge the emotional dimension related to them. Philosophers have often ignored this reality and reduced ethical decision-making to deductive reasoning procedures. There has been much criticism in contemporary moral philosophy against this emphasis, not least due to its perceived neglect of the importance of emotions in moral life. One of the earlier critics, Iris Murdoch, accused the whole Kantian tradition in moral philosophy of reducing all values to the autonomous human will, and thus leaving emotions out of the moral sphere. In Murdoch's view, moral agency is reduced to "the making of sensible choices and the giving of sensible and simple reasons. It is not seen as the activity of theorizing, imagining, or seeking for deeper insight."[20] Murdoch has, among others, attempted to formulate an alternative view of moral life. Love is a central concept in this view. It is seen as the most important virtue, and as such, a condition of any kind of moral life. By Murdoch's definition, "love is the perception of individuals. Love is the extremely difficult realisation that something other than oneself is real. Love … is the discovery of reality."[21] As with Kant, love is here an activity, although rather than beneficence, it is "perception," "realization," and "discovery." The moral point with this definition of love as an activity, however, is not that it can be posited as a duty, but that without such love all moral life, as well as moral improvement, would be impossible. Moral improvement is equated with improvement in one's capacity to love.

4. Conclusion

Our aim in this chapter was to examine the contents of parental obligations in procreative decision-making with a special reference to selective abortion. We introduced two different assentist positions regarding parenthood and the rights of fetuses. Common to both of these positions is a Kantian notion of duties that parents assume towards their children. The positions differ in that whereas Rhodes sees these duties as conditional, that is, the assumed duties do not apply if it turns out that the fetus is impaired, Vehmas has argued that the assuming of parental duties should be unconditional from the moment that parents decide to procreate. According to this position selective abortion is a violation of parental duties.

After explaining these positions, we set out to answer the question whether such an unconditional attitude towards one's children can be posited as a duty? This question was set in the frame of the ideal of an unconditional parental *love* since love is commonly considered as necessary for a positive and secure environment for children to grow in, and securing such an environment could be considered, if anything, one of parental duties. Thus, the question came to be whether there can be a duty to love one's children irrespective of the characteristics that they might have? From the perspective of a Kantian distinction between pathological and practical love it turned out that the kind of parental love commonly thought as essential to good parenthood cannot be posited as a duty. Now, what follows from this with respect to selective abortion?

First, it could follow that parents should terminate the pregnancy if the prenatal diagnosis discloses their future child to have the kind of condition that the parents could not accept; that is, if they would have the kind of child they could not learn to love wholeheartedly, they should, as responsible agents, choose selective abortion. The second option is to view parenthood as an unconditional position and thus accept *any* child with a prospect for a life worth living. If the thought of having a child with impairment appears difficult for parents, they should examine their emotional reactions and possible difficulties of relating to such a child. Then, they should try to correct the kind of prejudices that prevent them of developing love for their future disabled child and try to cultivate the kind of loving emotions and feelings that would enable them to *act and feel* as loving parents do.

There is always the possibility that parents fail to love and care for their (disabled or non-disabled) children properly. The project of cultivating one's feelings for one's child thus always includes the risk of failure, although empirical studies show that while parents are often shocked at first when having a child with impairment, in the course of time, they usually adapt both cognitively and emotionally to the situation. However, since the project of cultivating one's feelings is a very complicated process, the person most capable of evaluating the likelihood of its success is the parent herself. It seems fair to suppose that she is the one possessing most information concerning her own ideals, emotional habits, strengths and weaknesses.

Further, because parenting is such a complex personal project, it seems somewhat inappropriate to conceptualize parenthood and selective abortion solely in terms of a duty-based account. There are various intervening factors, particularities that make general norms questionable in this context. When parenting is seen from this angle, it would seem more appropriate to understand parenthood and selective abortion in terms of what virtuous or ideal parents would do. Parental responsibility could then perhaps be summed up as commitment to the improvement of one's capacity to love, rather than committing to any set of specific duties. This would also mean that moral agents themselves would have to work out the exact implications of their own parental ideals, that is, what is good or bad for them, and right or wrong regarding parenthood in general.

NOTES

1. Rosamond Rhodes, "Abortion and Assent," *Cambridge Quarterly of Healthcare Ethics*, 8 (1999), pp. 416–427.

2. Simo Vehmas, "Assent and Selective Abortion: A Response to Rhodes and Häyry," *Cambridge Quarterly of Healthcare Ethics*, 10 (2001), pp. 433–440; Simo Vehmas, "Parental Responsibility and the Morality of Selective Abortion," *Ethical Theory and Moral Practice*, 5 (2002), pp. 463–484; see also Adrienne Asch, "Why I Haven't Changed My Mind about Prenatal Diagnosis: Reflections and Refinements," *Prenatal Testing and Disability Rights*, ed. Erik Parens and Adrienne Asch (Washington, DC: Georgetown University Press, 2000), pp. 234–258; Marsha Saxton, "Why Members of the Disability Community Oppose Prenatal Diagnosis and Selective Abortion," *Prenatal Testing and Disability Rights*, pp. 147–164.

3. Rhodes, "Abortion and Assent," p. 417; Vehmas, "Parental Responsibility and the Morality of Selective Abortion," pp. 475–476.

4. Matti Häyry, "Abortion, Disability, Assent, and Consent," *Cambridge Quarterly of Healthcare Ethics*, 10 (2001), pp. 79–87.

5. See *e.g.* Marcia Baron, *Kantian Ethics Almost without Apology* (Ithaca: Cornell University Press, 1995); Paul Guyer, *Kant on Freedom, Law, and Happiness* (Cambridge: Cambridge University Press, 2000); Barbara Herman, *The Practice of Moral Judgment* (Cambridge: Harvard University Press, 1993); Kelly D. Sorensen, "Kant's Taxonomy of the Emotions," *Kantian Review*, 6 (2002), pp. 109–128.

6. Guyer, *Kant on Freedom, Law, and Happiness*, p. 299.

7. Immanuel Kant, *Anthropology from a Pragmatic Point of View*, trans. Mary Gregor (Hague: Martinus Nijhoff, 1798/1974), 7:251.

8. Sorensen, "Kant's Taxonomy of the Emotions," pp. 111, 114.

9. Immanuel Kant, "The Metaphysics of Morals," *The Cambridge Edition to the Works of Immanuel Kant, Practical Philosophy*, trans. Mary Gregor (Cambridge: Cambridge University Press), 6:401 (references are to the *Akademie* volume and page numbers).

10. *Ibid.*, 6:449.

11. *Ibid.*, 6:450.

12. Barbara P. Solheim, "The Possibility of a Duty to Love," *Journal of Social Philosophy*, 30 (1999), pp. 1–17.

13. *Ibid.*, p. 2.

14. *Ibid.*, p. 7.

15. Hugh LaFollette, *Personal Relationships: Love, Identity, and Morality* (Oxford: Blackwell, 1996), pp. 28–30, 34–35, 38–39.

16. *Cf.*, *e.g.*, Kant, *The Metaphysics of Morals*, 6:399–400; 6:402; 6:443.

17. LaFollette, *Personal Relationships*, pp. 32–34.

18. *Ibid.*, p. 35.

19. Solheim, "The Possibility of a Duty to Love," p. 10.

20. Iris Murdoch, "A House of Theory," *Existentialists and Mystics: Writings on Philosophy and Literature*, ed. Peter Conradi (New York: Penguin Books, 1958/1999), pp. 171–186, p. 177.

21. Iris Murdoch, "The Sublime and the Good," *Existentialists and Mystics: Writings on Philosophy and Literature*, ed. Peter Conradi (New York: Penguin Books, 1959/1999), pp. 205–220, p. 215.

Seventeen

THE MEANING OF SUFFERING: A CRITIQUE OF THE HÄYRY SYNDROME

Frank J. Leavitt

1. Introduction

Matti Häyry has suggested the term, "Prereproductive Stress Syndrome" for infertile couples who find themselves in stress and turn to fertility technology for a solution. The first researcher to identify and define a medical syndrome often gets immortalized by having the syndrome called after his or her name. I therefore suggest the term: *Häyry Syndrome.* In Matti's opinion, when Häyry Syndrome sufferers turn to fertility technology as a solution to their problem, they "could be told that, according to at least one philosopher, it would be all right for them not to reproduce at all."[1]

Matti has a number of reasons for his opinion, including argumentation based on some technical points in Professor Rawls' philosophy. But I want to cut through the technicalities and scholarly discussions. I want instead to get directly to the heart of Matti's opinion, which I believe is summed up in the following statement in his essay:

> I am also personally convinced that it is *immoral* to have children. Children can suffer, and I think it is wrong to bring about avoidable suffering. By deliberately having children parents enable suffering which could have been avoided by reproductive abstinence. This is why I believe that human procreation is fundamentally immoral.[2]

In a response, Søren Holm commented: "Few now hold the belief that an engagement with philosophy has strong therapeutic effects (even fewer when they have met real life philosophers)."[3] I share Søren's doubts of the value of quoting philosophers in clinical practice. Indeed I doubt that it is of much value for philosophers to work as "clinical ethicists," who may simply relieve the medical staff of responsibility for ethical decisions. Calling in an ethicist is an easy way to wash one's hands. But philosophers do have a role as educators. Many philosophers teach in medical schools. Physicians and future physicians can hear philosophers' opinions, weigh them against other opinions, and draw their own conclusions for clinical practice. It is for this reason that I think that a discussion of Matti's opinion may be of value not only for philosophical entertainment, but also for clinical practice.

In spite of the fact, which I shall presently explain, that Matti does not really believe that it is "wrong to bring about avoidable suffering," I think that the statement which I have just quoted expresses the heart of his opinion. And that is the statement which I shall discuss.

Actually, I am quite sympathetic to Matti's clinical conclusion that infertile couples can be advised that "it would be all right for them not to reproduce at all." But I disagree with Matti's reasons for his conclusion. I am, moreover, a happy father of five and a grandfather of five. I am a loyal member of a society where childbirth and large families are encouraged. I look forward to my unmarried children getting married: the sooner the better. And I look forward to all of my children having their own children: the more the better. But, for reasons other than Matti's, I agree that fertility technology is not necessarily the best option for couples who are not fortunate enough to have children in the natural way.

Incidentally, it is surprising that Matti, who believes that it is immoral to have children, should make fertility technology the main issue in his paper. Many, many more people have children through the traditional method. Indeed, fertility technology seems to be restricted to a tiny affluent minority. The issue of fertility technology may be statistically quite insignificant globally. I am surprised that, instead of attacking fertility technology, Matti doesn't make an all-out attack against reproduction in general, perhaps by writing polemics in favor of perpetual virginity. (Birth control would be out, because birth control can fail and Matti seems to oppose taking any risk, even statistically rather small risks, of causing suffering.) But since Matti has chosen to discuss fertility technology, I'll discuss it as well.

I'll explain in section 2 of this chapter why it is clear that Matti does not really believe what he says. This will lead, in section 3, to a discussion of the meaning of suffering. Finally, in section 4, I'll explain why I am sympathetic to Matti's clinical conclusion, even though I am all for having children.

2. How It Can Be Good to Bring About Avoidable Suffering

Not long ago I showed Matti a paper which I had written. He suggested that I submit it to a journal of which he is a sub-editor. At the same time he made some suggestions for revisions. Dutifully, I carried out his suggestions. Not writing or researching easily, I endured quite a bit of suffering as I toiled away to re-research and re-write the paper. Finally I thought that the paper was good enough for me to submit it proudly to Matti. But what did Matti do? He sent it to readers, got their criticisms, and sent me a whole bunch of further requests for revisions: thereby causing me even more suffering. In spite of all this torture, however, I thank Matti today. Of course he did the right thing to request revisions. Of course he did the right thing to send the paper to referees and then request more revisions. Matti's editorial sadism lead, I trust, to a better paper. And it lead to my learning quite a few things which I do not think I could have learned without that suffering.

I am not saying that all suffering which editors cause can lead to learning things. For example, when a publisher scorns academic and literary freedom and (rather than simply asking for consistency) insists on arbitrary standards of style and spelling, as well as linguistic adherence to a preconceived political ideology, about the only lesson which one learns is to submit in future to other publishers. But this rare example aside, I think that editorial sadism is usually benign.

The reader will object that this kind of suffering barely deserves the name of "suffering," so minor it is, as compared to the horrid and intense suffering which so many human beings have to endure. This is true, and the more horrid forms of suffering will be discussed later. But there is an important bioethical lesson to learn from even such a weak form of suffering. There is often a process, a causal relationship—which utilitarians often ignore—between suffering and good results.

Some excellent examples may be found in a book by the British physician, Sir George Pickering.[4] According to Pickering, Charles Darwin, Florence Nightingale and Mary Baker Eddy, among others, arrived at some of their most fruitful ideas while suffering from illness. Pickering observes that there may be a close connection between illness and creative thinking. Illness gives one time to reflect. One is, hopefully, relieved of the burdens of daily business. Illness provides an excellent excuse for neglecting tedious chores, and for keeping guests and family members away, so that one can concentrate on creative work.

About fifteen years ago, I was driving my car home after spending the day at a library in Jerusalem. In a suburb of Bethlehem, an Arab threw a stone at me. The combined force of the stone and my speeding car smashed half of my head. Unconscious, all of my weight was on the accelerator pedal and the car sped ahead. Fortunately a soldier hitchhiker grabbed the steering wheel, turned off the ignition, and guided the car to a safe stop, saving both of our lives. I endured a rather memorable amount of suffering as a result of this experience. But my suffering had beneficial results. Besides the benefits to the maxillo-facial surgeons, who gained valuable experience during the fourteen hours they spent reassembling my head, I also gained from the event. The experience made me more tolerant and accepting. Although we have a war with the stone thrower, and others like him, I do not hate them. They are doing what they have to do, and I am doing what I have to do. It also gave me something which some people would call faith, but which I would call a kind of metaphysical calmness inside. It made me more fearless in dangerous circumstances, and helped me to set an example to others not to give in to terrorists, and not to let them frighten us into not traveling freely.

Utilitarians and other philosophers may easily pass over this intimate relationship between suffering and beneficial effects. In a response to Matti, Bennett says, "as long as the suffering a life contains is likely to be outweighed by positive experiences, choosing to bring such a life into being is morally acceptable, even if the reasons for this choice are irrational." [5] This kind of cost accounting has its value. But it utterly misses the interesting details of the internal, causal processes which often lead from suffering to good.

3. The Meaning of Suffering

People who survived the Nazi holocaust, or the American atomic bombings of Hiroshima and Nagasaki, or whose children have been killed or permanently maimed and crippled in recent terror attacks, may accuse me of obscenity for daring to compare the victims of editorial sadism to the victims of real suffering. My own suffering from the head injury was infinitesimal as compared to what these people have endured. Their accusation would be quite justified. I gave the example of editorial sadism because it helps us to see that nobody, not even Matti, can be totally against all suffering. But much more importantly, editorial sadism gives us a simple way to understand the causal relationship which may hold between suffering and benefit.

There are, however, three major differences between real suffering and the suffering which is caused by editorial sadism or by my head injury. The first is the enormity of the suffering which individuals may endure. The second is the enormity of the numbers of people who may suffer in real suffering.

The third difference far surpasses our ability to make sense of human life. While editorial sadism and injuries like my own can and often do result in clear benefit, real suffering often seems to benefit nobody. A Hiroshima housewife, who had nothing to do with the bombing of Pearl Harbor, was on her way to buy groceries. Suddenly she was walking around with burning flesh falling from her skeleton. For what? People suffer, are miserable, die, and that is the end of it. But why should I make my weak attempts at eloquence when Shakespeare's Macbeth has said it all:

> Life's but a walking shadow, a poor player
> That struts and frets his hour upon the stage
> And then is heard no more: it is a tale
> Told by an idiot, full of sound and fury,
> Signifying nothing.

Religions say they have an answer: Suffering which we endure in this life may sometimes be rewarded in this life. But when it isn't, then its purpose is to prepare us for another life, or at least for another state, or other states, of existence.

According to a Christian version of the religious answer, the suffering which we endure in this life may be deducted from the account of the punishments for our sins, which await us in the next life. The more we suffer now, the less we'll have to suffer in Hell or Purgatory.

Mystical Judaism (kabala) and Hinduism have a more sophisticated answer which, to my mind, is easier to believe. I refer to the doctrine of reincarnation. Through suffering in each of many lives, we learn lessons: our souls become "repaired" or purified. Eventually, after enough lives and enough lessons and repairs (maybe millions) our souls will be fit for a blessed, spiritual state which requires no more incarnations.

Unlike mystical Judaism and Hinduism however, which see a meaning in our suffering, Buddhism says that our suffering is meaningless, as is all human life. But once one realizes the meaninglessness of life, one is freed from caring about it, and one reaches the Buddha nature, the state of eternal enlightenment in which no further incarnations are necessary. Macbeth and some existentialists resemble Buddhists to some extent, although they lack the state of eternal enlightenment.

Can any of these doctrines be proved? In our private lives we may believe as we please. But as responsible university lecturers, we have a responsibility to base our opinions upon evidence and/or logical deduction. Personally I believe that I have had experiences in my life which only a doctrine of reincarnation seems to provide a theoretical framework for explaining them. But I doubt that an account of such experiences would make much sense to anyone who has not had similar ones. So I'll leave them out of this paper. And I'll assume that none of these religious doctrines can be proved.

But the fact that they cannot be proved doesn't make them false. Indeed, there is neither adequate evidence to prove them, nor adequate evidence to disprove them. Among the three positions—theism, atheism and agnosticism—the only one which is "rational" in a philosophical or scientific sense is agnosticism. Only agnosticism does not require a blind leap of faith. It takes a great deal of faith to state with bold certitude that God or afterlives do not exist. How can anyone possibly know this? Some people think that they can prove that God does not exist by arguing that an all-powerful, all-good God could or would not create so much suffering. But Judaism does not teach that God is all-good. Judaism teaches that we should bless God both for the good and for the bad. So although this argument might work against the Christian God, it doesn't work against the God of Israel.

The fact is that we do not and cannot know anything at all about the meaning of life, if it has a meaning, or about the meaning of suffering, if it has a meaning.

But if we do not know what if any meaning suffering has, then we have no grounds to draw philosophical conclusions from our ideas about it. And we have, *a fortiori,* no grounds to draw conclusions for clinical medicine. Not knowing what happens to people after death, we have no way to even guess whether bringing these people into existence is a good thing or a bad thing. Of course anyone who is born has a good chance of suffering. But we have no way to tell whether or not this suffering will lead to greater goods for them. So, in cases where our suffering does not lead to clear benefits in this life, we have no foundations for either agreeing or for disagreeing with Matti's opinion that it is unethical to bring about avoidable suffering.

Sahin Aksoy based his disagreement with Matti on his opinion that: "life and existence is always better than non-existence."[6] But we cannot know anything about this subject either. "Non-existence" can either mean *non-existence in this world*, or it can mean *absolute non-existence.* If the former is meant, then we really have no way of knowing which is better. For if souls which are not born into this world exist in some other world, we do not know whether existence in that other world is a paradise or a hell or maybe even something else which goes far beyond our powers of imagination and speech. But absolute non-existence cannot enter into our consideration either because we have no way of knowing whether souls which do not exist in this world exist in some other world or absolutely don't exist. There is, therefore, no way to know whether Sahin's opinion is true or false. So it is clinically irrelevant.

In a reply to Sahin, Matti has asked: "Who exactly is the absent someone who is sentenced to non-existence; and who precisely is the unborn child whose interests would be served by bringing her to birth? How can we attribute experiences and interests to beings who have not existed in the past, do not exist now, and will possibly never exist in the future?"[7]

I assume that Matti's rhetorical questions are not quite about *unborn* children, who may exist *in utero,* but about children who have not yet been conceived. But if Matti thinks that as-yet not conceived children do not exist in any way, shape or form, I will not state dogmatically that Matti is wrong. I will only state that it is dogmatic to take any stand on this issue. Maybe before we were conceived we existed in other bodies; maybe we existed as unembodied souls; maybe we existed in some form which we are incapable of conceiving; and maybe Matti is right and we didn't exist in any way, shape or form. All we can say is that we do not know.

Indeed, assuming that it is likely that anyone who is born will endure some suffering, we have no way of knowing whether or not this suffering would be avoided by not causing this person to be born. The reason is that some religious people would say that if we do not cause this soul to be born now, it will likely be born at another time and in other circumstances. And we have no way of predicting what its life would be like in the other time and circumstances.

Again, I am not saying that these religious views of life and suffering are true. But I am saying that we should not ignore the possibility that they might be true. I side with those people who—although not unaware of the likelihood that any child born may have to endure some degree of suffering in the course of a lifetime—proceed to have children in the calm optimism, that no matter what suffering may await human beings, all will be well in the end. This calm optimism, which is one of the benefits I received from my head injury, described above, is too easily confused with what some religious people call "faith." But "faith" has too many connotations of uncritical, brainwashed religious fanaticisms of various kinds. So I prefer to talk not about faith but about calm optimism instead.

4. In Favor of Children, But Not so Sure About Reproductive Technology

As I have mentioned, I am all for having children. My main reason is a simple, non-philosophical love of children and life. I am glad I live in a society where this love is shared. As I have already explained, Matti's arguments about suffering do not impress me. There are other arguments, better known than Matti's, against having children. These arguments are based on the assumption that the earth can no longer support human population growth. These arguments do not impress me either. In the first place, while we talk about global overcrowding, factors tending to reduce human population can always surprise us. We have the AIDS pandemic which is tragically reducing African population and may do the same elsewhere. We have Tsunamis, hurricanes and earthquakes. A few years ago, Islamic terrorists reduced U.S. population by more than 3000 in one day, and they seem to be planning even more extravagant shows. I am not so sure that birth control is at all needed to reverse human population growth.

In the second place, while some people look at the overcrowded parts of the world, I tend to look at the empty places. Flying over eastern Russia on my way from Japan to Europe I am astonished at the seemingly infinite expanses of greenery and torrential rivers. The earth has plenty of land and water for all. One should also think of the unused deserts of the Earth: Saudi Arabia, the Sinai, North Africa and more. My own country, Israel, was highly fertile in Biblical times. But in the thousands of years of our exile, it was turned into desert by the uncontrolled and unintelligent grazing of sheep and goats. After the revival of Zionism on a significant scale about a hundred years ago, the desert has become green again through hard work, intelligent agricultural technology and innovation. More recently, during the fifteen years, from 1967 to 1982, during which we held the northern Sinai, we turned the sterile sand dunes of that area into highly fertile agricultural land. Digging under the surface of the sand, one could even see black streaks, signs of the beginnings of organic soil created by the rotting roots of our previous crops. After we agreed to give the Sinai to Egypt, however, and during the last few days before our withdrawal, Bedouin tribesmen arrived on camels, herding huge flocks of sheep and goats. They quickly devastated our remaining greenery, returning the land once more to desert. But the fact remains that we have proved that sterile deserts can be turned green. Handling shifting dune sand is not easy.[8] But difficulties are not insurmountable. The earth has the agricultural potential for much more population growth.

As I've also mentioned, however, I do not totally disagree with Matti's proposal that when Häyry Syndrome couples turn to fertility technology as a solution to their problem, they could be told that it would be all right for them not to reproduce at all. I would like to modify his proposal, however, and would like to propose instead that various alternatives to fertility technology be explained. One alternative is not reproducing, but adopting a baby instead. Other alternatives are natural, traditional, non-technological ways in which an infertile couple can have a baby. These will be explained presently.

I do not know how many people working in fertility clinics would be willing to suggest alternatives. Entire medical professions and infrastructures get built up over new technologies. It is hard to shake them once they exist. But I do think it would be worthwhile if such couples could be persuaded to think of other alternatives. I have three reasons for believing this.

In the first place, although many questions are being asked nowadays about the ethics of high-tech fertility, intracytoplasmic sperm injection, human reproductive cloning, and the like, these questions are coming too late. These questions should have been asked when human artificial insemination was first tried, because it was such a radical departure from the traditional way of making babies. In most, although perhaps not all, societies, religion, legend and culture have always assumed that we all have or have had fathers in the traditional sense of the word: a man who got one's mother pregnant in the old way of getting women pregnant. Freud and other psychoanalysts wrote about the impact on our personalities of our relationship with the man who fathered us in the traditional sense. What will be the personalities of people who do not have fathers in this sense? What, moreover, is it like to be conceived in the impersonal environment of laboratory equipment, as compared to the warm contact of human bodies? I am not saying that fertility technology is detrimental to the child. I am only saying that we do not know. I am very happy for friends and neighbors who delight in their IVF children. But citing a few examples of wonderful IVF children is inadequate evidence for medical science, which is trying to become evidence-based. Most parents of IVF babies seem to disappear with no researched follow-up being carried out. We need very long-term longitudinal studies over very large populations. Some such studies have been published. But it is too early to draw any general conclusions. In the meantime, and with all due respect to my friends who have IVF children, and to my colleagues who work in IVF from a sincere desire to help people, I cannot be a supporter of IVF.

In the second place, ancient societies have had other means of coping with infertility. Here in Israel we have the Biblical example of Rachel and Ya-akov (Jacob). As many readers will recall, Yaakov married two sisters, Leah and Rachel. He and Leah had children. But Rachel was unable to get pregnant. The Bible tells (in the King James Version):

> And when Rachel saw that she bare Jacob no children, Rachel envied her sister; and said unto Jacob, Give me children, or else I die. And Jacob's anger was kindled against Rachel: and he said, Am I in God's stead, who hath withheld from thee the fruit of the womb? And she said, Behold my maid Bilhah, go in unto her; and she shall bear upon my knees that I may also have children by her. And she gave him Bilhah her handmaid to wife: and Jacob went in unto her. And Bilhah conceived, and bare Jacob a son. (Genesis XXX, 1-5)

Later on, with the help of a herbal treatment, Rachel bore two children herself, Yosef and Binyamin, dying during the second childbirth. But this is besides our present point. Yaakov and Rachel are considered very holy people by Jews and other Bible-believing peoples. When a couple's infertility seems to be due to a problem with the wife, Bible-believing religious leaders should urge them to consider following the example of Yaakov and Leah and allowing the husband to have babies through another woman, rather than turning to fertility technology.

For cases where a couple's infertility seems to be due to a problem with the husband, the Japanese used to have a solution. In Ibaraki Prefecture not far from Tokyo and near the science and university city of Tsukuba, there is a holy mountain called *Tsukuba-san* (Mount Tsukuba). *Tsukuba-san* has two peaks representing the male and female deities, Isanage and Isanami, who are said to have created the islands of Japan. The mountain is connected with fertility in Shinto belief, and one often sees there pairs of stones, one tall and thin and the other low, round and with a crack: representing the male and the female. I once visited a spot on *Tsukuba-san* where annual bacchanalian free-love festivals were held from ancient times until they were stopped in the modern age. People would come from all over Japan for the festival. A Shinto priest told me: "It was an excellent solution for infertile couples."

Today, it would be hard to gain acceptance for this kind of solution among many religions, especially those that accept the Bible, in which the prohibition of sex with a married woman is very strong. Two of the Ten Commandments relate to this prohibition. Religions, however, can be pretty ingenious in time of need, and can sometimes find ways to get around divine prohibitions. Perhaps the idea should be considered as an alternative to fertility technology.

In the third place, I wonder how often adoption is seriously considered as an alternative to fertility technology. War, disaster and disease have created so many orphans in the world; it is a shame that more infertile couples are not considering this solution. It is also a shame that so many resources are invested in high-tech solutions rather than in building logistic and support infrastructures to make it easier to adopt babies from poor countries, war zones, and disaster areas.

On the other hand, since my wife and I have been lucky with children, I cannot judge those couples who insist upon having their own children through fertility technology. I would not have the heart to argue with them. But I do think that alternatives might be gently suggested.

NOTES

1. Matti Häyry, "A Rational Cure for Prereproductive Stress Syndrome," *Journal of Medical Ethics*, 30 (2004), pp. 377–378.

2. Häyry, "A rational cure for prereproductive stress syndrome," p. 377.

3. Søren Holm, "Why It Is Not Strongly Irrational to Have Children," *Journal of Medical Ethics*, 30 (2004), p. 381.

4. George Pickering, *Creative Malady* (New York, Oxford University Press, 1974).

5. Rebecca Bennett, "Human Reproduction: Irrational But in Most Cases Morally Defensible," *Journal of Medical Ethics*, 30 (2004), pp. 379–380.

6. Sahin Aksoy, "Response to: A Rational Cure for Pre-Reproductive Stress Syndrome," *Journal of Medical Ethics*, 30 (2004), pp. 382–383.

7. Matti Häyry, "The Rational Cure for Prereproductive Stress Syndrome Revisited," *Journal of Medical Ethics*, 31 (2005), pp. 606–607.

8. Frank J. Leavitt, "Making the Desert Bloom," (correspondence) *Nature*, 19 (1993), p. 366.

Eighteen

IS IT IRRATIONAL TO HAVE CHILDREN?

Richard Ashcroft

1. Matti Häyry's Argument

Matti Häyry has advanced what he takes to be a knock-down argument against the rationality of child-bearing for *everyone*. It goes like this:

> I am convinced it is *irrational* to have children. This conviction is based on two beliefs that I hold. I believe it would be irrational to choose the course of action that can realistically lead to the worst possible outcome. And I believe that having a child can always realistically lead to the worst possible outcome, when the alternative is not to have a child.[1]

He also has a version concerning the immorality of having children:

> I am also personally convinced that it is *immoral* to have children. Children can suffer, and I think it is wrong to bring about avoidable suffering. By deliberately having children parents enable suffering which could have been avoided by reproductive abstinence. This is why I believe that human procreation is fundamentally immoral.[2]

I will not here address the immorality argument, which turns on fundamentally the same conceptions of formal argument and of causation, outcome, comparison between suffering and non-existence. The issue of the relationship between the rational and the moral is too complex to go into here. Here I am interested in the questions of rationality raised by this argument.

Before we go any further, it is worth setting this argument into the context of Matti Häyry's previous work. One interpretation might go as follows: in this paper (and in his reply to critics[3]) he is simply drawing a logical conclusion from a previous paper[4] in which he argued that it is both irrational and immoral to bear children who are at risk of perinatal infection by the mother with HIV. In fact in this paper, he conflates the rational and the moral, as (some) consequentialists often do. Here is what he says:

The normative starting point of this paper is simply that avoidable suffering should not be inflicted, by acts or omissions, on actual or prospective individuals, unless even greater suffering can thereby be alleviated or prevented. This is a position I share with many contemporary philosophers of the consequentialist tradition.[5]

In this earlier paper (first presented in 1995) he concentrates on the policy options for preventing, or reducing the number of, births of HIV positive babies, taking it as given that to be born HIV positive is to be born harmed. He then generalizes to other kinds of disorder, disease or disability:

> I agree that it would be wrong to single out HIV carriers, and blame only them for bringing suffering children into existence. I do not however, wish to restrict my comments to them. Everybody who intentionally or negligently allows avoidable suffering in reproductive matters is equally guilty, be the source of suffering medical, social or hereditary.[6]

The relevant difference between the argument in 1995 and the argument of 2004-5 is that in 1995 he was comparing the state of children born with HIV with that of children born without (other things being equal), whereas in 2004-5 he was comparing the state of children born with the state of non-existence (if state it be). Notwithstanding the notorious difficulties involved in comparing the state of existence with the (non-)state of non-existence, or in comparing children born in different possible worlds with different characteristics,[7] many people would want to say that a child is harmed in some relatively commonsense terms if it is born HIV positive, and this could have been avoided. As Matti Häyry says in his 2004 article:

> The conclusion relies on the judgement that human lives can sometimes be bad. Individuals who see their own lives as good, and assert that everybody else's life must be similarly assessed have frequently challenged this view. Many actual people believe, however, that they would have been better off had they not been born. This is often the essence of "wrongful life" charges on which individuals have sued their parents or medical providers for damages. These legal claims may be controversial, but it cannot be disputed that at least some of the people in question genuinely see their lives as worse than non-existence.[8]

Now in recent work Julian Savulescu has applied consequentialist reasoning consistent with Matti Häyry's 1995 argument to ground a principle of procreative beneficence, such that would-be parents are obliged to ensure that any child they bring into being is as well off genetically and environmentally as they can manage. Crudely put, to do less than this is to harm the infant, since there is, relative to these parents, a possible infant in comparison to whom this actual infant is worse off.[9] This, if you like, is the "positive utilitarian" version of what Matti Häyry is attempting in "negative utilitarian" guise in 1995 and in 2004-5. I must confess that I feel more comfortable, metaphysically, with the positive utilitarian version of the argument, since we are comparing identifiable individuals and their measurable welfare, albeit across distinct logically possible worlds, rather than individuals with non-individuals.[10] Nonetheless, I do not feel that this is the interesting element in the argument here. Intuitively, we do make such comparisons, although we may be wrong to do so; theoretically, there may be ways to reconstruct our intuitions appropriately in order to make nearly equivalent comparisons. But the power of Matti Häyry's argument lies with its claim to *rationality* rather than any more or less debatable metaphysical or epistemological claims about the substantive matter of possible comparison. In this I think at least Bennett and Aksoy partially miss the point.

Before we leave this question of negative or positive utilitarianism, it is interesting to recall what Matti Häyry said about this issue in his major theoretical statement, *Liberal Utilitarianism and Applied Ethics* (1994):

> An axiological variant which is closely related to the "need" and "interest" approaches is "negative utilitarianism," which states that it is not the maximization of pleasure but the minimization of pain that counts in the moral assessment of actions. ... [I]t can be argued that the most effective way to minimize suffering in the world would be the extinction of all sentient life forms. But nihilist normative conclusions like this are widely regarded as immoral.[11]

Later he argues that, on his own needs-based reconstruction of utilitarianism, this "negatively hedonistic strategy" would be blocked:

> Since many sentient beings recognize in themselves a need to survive and a need to make autonomous choices concerning their own lives, the principles of liberal utilitarianism would not condone the minimization of suffering by minimizing the number of beings who have the capacity to suffer.[12]

Indeed, at this point he allows that "even granting that the removal of pain and misery is more urgent than the promotion of positive happiness, it cannot be denied that it is the latter that provides life with its ultimate value."[13] This qualification is surprising in the light of the position he reaches in 1999, in an essay investigating the normative and axiological foundations of John Harris's work in applied ethics:

> Although the fully voluntary extinction of humankind ought to be condoned, there will, one could argue, always be people who want the human race to continue to exist. As these individuals cannot legitimately be forced to cooperate, the extinction must presumably be condemned.[14]

Here he admits that one can assume "that individuals can have a serious need to have their own children". Given that his own liberal utilitarianism has as an axiom the following:

> *The principle of other-regarding need frustration*
> When the need satisfaction produced by various action alternatives is assessed, the most basic needs of one individual or group shall be considered only if the satisfaction of those needs does not frustrate the needs of others at the same hierarchical level.[15]

This is hardly surprising, but what is clear is that for Häyry although we may be barred from compelling others to adopt this pain minimization strategy (of non-reproduction) by this principle, we are fully entitled to talk them out of it. Hence, in 1995, he argues that firm social disapproval is a legitimate tool of persuasion to discourage HIV positive women from having children at significant risk of HIV infection, and in 2004-5, he says:

> I am fully aware that other people have different moral views on this and other matters. I do not think moral considerations are universal, overriding commands, as some philosophers do. I think they are opinions which I am entitled to express freely in private and in public, as I think other people should be entitled to express their opinions.[16]

While in 1999 there is an ambiguous note to his suggestion that voluntary extinction be "condoned", as it is in the context of whether *John Harris's* views about the impermissibility of voluntary extinction are consistent with *John Harris's* negative utilitarian views (as Häyry sees them), by 2004 the ambiguity has passed, and Häyry is advocating quite explicitly a voluntary extinctionist position. This seems to involve a retreat from his 1994 view that positive pleasure was of legitimate interest to the utilitarian and analytically distinct from the simple absence of pain or suffering. In retrospect, his admirably liberal and humane, dare I say Enlightenment, version of utilitarianism of 1994 has now been fully driven out by a Schopenhauerian version of utilitarianism, in which the only reason not to annihilate the human race (and other sentient creatures) is that doing so *coercively* would create even more anguish, through the violation of autonomy and the frustration of certain basic, if irrational, needs.

2. Defeating Häyry's Argument

Having set out Matti Häyry's argument for the irrationality of procreation, I have set it into the context of his work on utilitarianism and its applications. I think grounding it in his previous work on "wrongful life" due to foreseeable medical or genetic harms or wrongs to future people shows something of the point of the argument, as well as illustrating its structure more perspicuously. But of course the argument is a formal one, standing on its own feet, and although this contextualising work may help orient the mind, we should perhaps disregard it in evaluating the argument.

Other commentators have suggested two lines of attack. The first is to dispute that the form of rationality Häyry has taken to be normative in decision situations of this kind is in fact inapt to this sort of choice.[17] The second is to dispute Häyry's axiology.[18] According to the first line of attack, Häyry's approach to rationality is no more or less than the *precautionary principle*, which, it is argued, is not normative for rational choice and fails to be action-guiding in any useful way.[19] I find this entirely convincing. Although Häyry in his 2005 paper[20] denies that he takes it to be the *only* criterion of rationality, it is clear that sometimes[21] this is the criterion he is using to mount this argument. However, I don't find this argument against what Frank Jackson calls "decision-theoretic consequentialism" entirely conclusive, since something structurally very like this kind of rationality is at work in many (most?) commonsense decisions and choices, and so if it fails in this kind of low risk (but serious consequence?) situation, it is probably the axiology that is at fault, rather than the criterion of normative formal rationality.[22] An alternative, which I shall explore, would be to say that this kind of rationality is not rationality *tout court* but only a specific model of rationality embedded within a more general model. Häyry, in his reply to his critics[23] accepts this possibility, without acknowledging that this means that failure to adhere to the requirements of this decision-theoretic rationality is not in itself *irrationality tout court*.

Suppose, then, that we grant the possibility that decision-theoretic rationality just is rationality *tout court*. Suppose further that we accept (*pace* Bennett and Aksoy) Häyry's axiology, and in particular his proposals for the comparability of welfare between states of existence and inexistence of persons. And suppose, finally, that we accept that within decision-theoretic rationality is embedded (at least) classical first order propositional calculus, so that we are allowed to draw standard inferences from combinations of propositions. Then it does look as if we are committed to accepting Häyry's argument for the irrationality of procreation.

One way to block the argument, for those who accept his more obviously persuasive argument that it would be wrong to expose a foetus to a serious risk of HIV infection perinatally, would be to deny that existence (and any associated suffering) is formally comparable, in all cases, to existence with HIV. We could say: existence does involve some suffering, arguably as a necessary constituent of life. We could try to run an argument that such suffering, while bad in itself, is part of what constitutes the good life, considered as an "organic unity."[24] All things considered, although there are some organic unities which are overall bad, such as an infant life HIV positive and without access to treatment (perhaps), most are not. We can distinguish between a life with some suffering in it, from a life of suffering, and indeed a significant part of moral philosophy is devoted to doing just this and explaining how it can be done. However, Häyry may reasonably respond that his axiology does not permit this move, and that the distinction drawn misses the point that suffering, if bad, is bad and to be avoided even when the good things and experiences of life predominate. So we cannot pursue this line of argument while accepting his axiology.

Another approach might be to deny that we "allow" avoidable suffering by procreation. We might say that it is a foreseen, but not intended, consequence of an act whose intended consequence is a life of flourishing and value. Only where this act cannot reasonably be expected to have this good consequence, and where the foreseeable bad consequences cannot be minimized below the point where they outweigh flourishing or pleasure, should we desist from procreation. This is a "double effect" argument. However, given the uncertainty of the positive outcome of a procreative decision, it is hard to see that this helps much, on Häyry's premises. It does not appear to preserve our intuitions in the HIV case, since it allows one to reject that argument as much as the general argument.

3. Why Kill Time (When You Can Kill Yourself)[25]

I believe that Häyry's (apparent) extinctionism gives us a clue to the way out here. On Häyry's argument, we have a rational argument for suicide. Indeed, a strong rational argument (since it seems to make suicide rationally required, rather than only rationally permissible). For if "it would be irrational to choose the course of action which can realistically lead to the worst possible outcome", this means that continuing to live is irrational. I have no reason to suppose that tomorrow I will not be violently waylaid by gangsters or terrorists, subjected to horrible violence and humiliation, and left to a life of self-loathing and bodily agony. Continuing to live leaves this possibility perpetually open, and the way the world is going appears to involve the probability of this outcome rising.

It might be objected that *my* continuing to exist and procreation affect different people. And so they do. But perhaps not in a morally important way. If it is states of suffering with which we are concerned, it really doesn't matter who is in that state, and whether that state is a state of my future self, or of some other future self. We are not here concerned directly with morality (where we might distinguish between harming oneself and harming another) but with rationality, and the principle of avoidance of the worst possible outcome of decision-making, judged non-morally.

And yet I continue to live, and I hope so does Matti, for many years to come, other things being equal.

4. From Suicide to Procreation

French-Algerian writer Albert Camus famously explored the absurdity of continuing to live in his *The Myth of Sisyphus*. This theme has been explored insufficiently in English-language bioethics. The application of this thought here suggests a variety of responses to the irrationality of procreation argument. One obvious observation is that it shows that there is *nothing* specific to procreation in the irrationality argument, other than filling in Φ with "procreate" in the following argument schema:

> To choose a course of action that can realistically lead to the worst possible outcome is irrational
> To Φ is to choose a course of action that can realistically lead to the worst possible outcome
> *Therefore*, to Φ is irrational.

The very generality of this schema suggests that we are in trouble, since it is hard to conceive of an action to specify Φ which does not make good semantic sense of the schema. As noted above, part of the problem may be with the semantics of "realistically lead to the worst possible outcome." Following on from this thought, we might reasonably argue about whether to ascribe this characteristic to actions is not really to pick out any morally relevant features of the action (if we allow that any action can go wrong), and indeed need not be the "privileged" description of the action in question. Indeed, we might say that to say of an act that it can go wrong is merely to say that it is an *act*. It seems at least superficially plausible that the capacity to misfire or generate unintended consequences is a necessary feature of action *per se*. So concentration of this feature of actions does not pick out which actions are to be preferred or dispreferred.

This argument is attractive, but has all the advantages of "theft over honest toil." We do after all characterize some acts as reckless or negligent, and hence *more* likely to misfire than actions which are not reckless or negligent. Here all Häyry needs to show is that of the option set {*procreate, don't procreate*}, *procreate* is more likely to misfire than *don't procreate*. Note in passing that as a consistent utilitarian, Häyry's theory of action includes a denial of the act/omission distinction, so that the given option set is a set of actions which are comparable, rather than the murkier comparison between acting and not acting. What he does not deny, however, is the existence/non-existence distinction, so that there is a genuine difference between *continue to exist* and *don't continue to exist*.

While I think there is some mileage in the semantic argument, I will not pursue it here, as it takes us too deeply into the theory of action and the theory of descriptions.[26] Another approach would be to argue that the no-procreation-suicide-instead result is a *reductio ad absurdum* of the argument schema. Thus, although we cannot show that the schema leads to a strict contradiction, no "reasonable person" would accept in informal reasoning a set of premises entailing such a conclusion. Were it not for the consistency of Häyry's argumentation over the past 10 years and the fact that he has published versions of this argument several times, and rebuttals of criticisms of this argument, one could even think that he *intended* the argument to be taken as a *reductio*. But I think this unlikely. It is, however, clear that this *reductio* was foreseen in his 1994 thoughts on the problems of negative utilitarianism, even though since 1994 he has changed its mind about whether it is *ad absurdum*.

We might be somewhat more generous, and argue that there is in fact *nothing* wrong with Häyry's argument here, and that the validity of his argument scheme and apparent acceptability of his premises entails that the argument is sound. Thus, he (with our help) has established an antinomy of practical reason. This is, in its turn, a conclusion supporting a sort of *absurdist* approach to living and procreating. We can neither justify these activities, nor their rejection. We simply choose, beyond reason. There may be a dialectical argument which grounds a particular resolution of the antinomies, but there will always be something fishy about this resolution.

So, our tour around Häyry's arguments may lead us to the following conclusion:

> The choice to procreate cannot be justified consistently with decision-theoretic consequentialism and its embedded rationality. But neither is it irrational. The decision is thus a pure choice.

5. Rationality and Procreation, Revisited

I showed how Häyry's argument could be understood as a generalization of an argument against bearing children subject to actual or probable serious medical or genetic disorder or disability. I then showed how the general argument, if taken in full generality, amounted to an argument for a rational requirement to commit suicide. I reviewed various ways to block this argument. The most natural, I concluded, was that we take the argument not to establish the irrationality of procreation, but instead the existential absurdity of both procreation and non-procreation.

In a sense this is a cheering result. It shows—if correct—that while it is not rational to have children, neither is it irrational, and this is an example of a domain of human freedom not bound by rational necessity.[27] And in one sense, this is coherent with an understanding of child-rearing as an assertion of human creativity and liberty in self-fashioning. However, I think that although this argument gives us a clue to how we should reason about procreation, it is incorrect as it stands.

An unsettling feature of Häyry's argument is that it does draw on one sort of reason *against* procreation, or at any rate for caution in procreation, which is acknowledged widely, viz., that to bring some kinds of children into the world, or to bring children into the world under some circumstances, is inadvisable where there is an alternative. A mistake in Häyry's approach is to exaggerate the force of reasons which may apply in some specific circumstances by taking them to give a categorical argument against procreation as such.

6. From Rationality Back to Reasons

In my discussion of Holm's critique of Häyry's reliance on the precautionary principle, I suggested that the rationality of decision-theoretic consequentialism could be embedded in rationality *tout court*. By this I meant that although for some purposes decision-theoretic consequentialism did indeed give normative criteria for decision-making, this was not in general the case. Some kinds of decision-making subject to reasons are not appropriately modelled by decision-theoretic consequentialism.[28] Consider first what Häyry's rational argument took for its premises—statements about beliefs. It was because it involved statements about beliefs that he was able, uncontroversially, to set out his argument as a syllogism. The next stage in his argument was to give accounts of why we should share the beliefs he laid down as premises in the syllogism. This is then purely an argument within theoretical reason. Now, in addition to theoretical reason, we have practical reason, which concerns normative reasons for action: what we ought to do, given what we want (and any moral motivations we may have). On the standard belief-desire model of philosophical psychology, it is clear that although beliefs about states of affairs should follow the norms of theoretical reasoning, it need not be the case that reasons for action have this structural constraint. As John Broome puts it, we *weigh* reasons:

> Intuitively, weighing is characteristic of goods. When we judge which of two options is better, we typically think that each option has some good and some bad features, which have to be weighed against each other. So we can use weighing as a criterion for what counts intuitively as a good. It is not the right criterion for the purposes of a theoretical account of

good. A theoretical account of good might allow one good to dominate another lexically, which rules out weighing.[29]

In the Häyry argument for the irrationality of procreation, it is assumed that some sort of domination *should* apply, which permits the risk aversion written into his account of decision-theoretic consequentialism not merely to be something shared by some to a greater or lesser extent, but actually to be normative for everyone.[30] The badness of suffering lexically dominates the goodness of other features of existence, albeit through the veil of uncertainty.

A second feature of practical reasoning and its structure is that it need not be subject to the law of excluded middle. If I have an option set with two members, of which only one can be realized, it need not be the case that practical reason tells me which I should realize. Suppose I live in a country where Sibling's Day is celebrated every year, and it is traditional to visit your siblings on that day. Suppose I have two brothers, equally dear to me, with whom I am on equally good terms. Sadly, they are not on good terms with each other, due to a failure on the part of one brother to visit the other one Sibling's Day a few years ago. Recently, they moved to opposite ends of our (very large) country, and it is no longer possible to visit both within 24 hours. Pick a brother. I have good reason to visit him, so I ought to do so, other things being equal. However, by permutation of the options, I have equally good reason to visit the other, other things being equal. I cannot visit both within 24 hours, and neither is willing to visit me since they are unwilling to risk meeting each other. It would be unthinkable for me not to visit at least one brother. My reason to visit either brother does not contradict my reason to visit the other. Some further reason is required to motivate my choice of which brother to visit.

Another feature of practical reason is that it involves reasoning on the basis of desires that I have. Such desires need not be consistent; my preferences may not be coherent. Internal conflict of desires is familiar to us all, and although some philosophers do argue that desires can be rationally corrected, it is part of the phenomenology of desire that changing or moderating one's desires, or resolving conflicts between desires, is difficult and painful. This suggests two things: first, that the structure of practical reason, to the extent that it reflects the structure of my desires, need not be particularly tidy. Second, the relationship between desires and reasons for action will be in part causal rather than rational. What I desire may cause me to desire it; that I desire something may cause me to see something as a reason for acting; what I take to be a reason for acting may, sometimes, alter my desires. In a sense this is why practical reason is considered practical—it relates to the operations of the mind and will in a world in which we are bodied forth as agents.

The theory of practical reason is an enormously complex and challenging field, in which much contemporary work in philosophy is being done. I hope I have done enough to motivate the thought that if the sort of rationality with which we are concerned in making decisions to procreate is practical reason, then some of the theoretically rational arguments proposed by Häyry may be misleading. It can, for instance, be rational in the present sense to weigh the options concerning procreation and decide in its favor. It can, further, be the case that factors like the desire to procreate, the desire to nurture and cherish a child or children, and the desire to give of oneself in this particular way are not simply reasons for action in the motivating sense (that agents' decisions to procreate can be explained by determining that these reasons are operative for them) but also in the normative sense—that they are good reasons for action, in that they are recognizable by the agent as giving sufficient reason to go on with their procreative and family-founding projects, and can be shared by others as such in judging the behavior of the would-be parents.

7. A Little Viennese Common Sense

I think we should consider the giving of reasons for (not) having children in Wittgensteinian terms: it may be that the question "why do you want to have children" makes no sense, or, that if it does, the answer "because I want to" is, as Wittgenstein said of some explanations, "where the spade turns." This is not to say that we cannot give further articulation to the reasons involved, if the person we are talking to appears not to understand. But in a rather profound sense, if this interlocutor keeps insisting on being given further grounds, or denies that the descriptions of the kinds of interests and emotions motivating one to want to procreate give accounts of *reasons*, then we are entitled to ask whether they have understood what is being said. It is not required of this account that the interlocutor shares these reasons or takes them to be reasons which should motivate him or her. But it is a requirement of mastery of the conceptual resources of English that they can see them *as* reasons.

The practice of giving reasons in dialogue is complex. One kind of reason-giving is contrastive: ordinarily in such a case we would do X, but we are here going to do Y—here's the reason. Outside a teaching situation, we would ordinarily not give reasons for each and every performance we undertake. In the case of procreation, the practice has changed from the expectation that reasons be given for *not* procreating to expecting that reasons be given *for* procreating. So be it. But let's not imagine that the reasons we are given for procreating *are not reasons at all*. Nor that these reasons are irrational, and the choice to act on them is, *ipso facto*, not irrational. To do that, adapting Wittgenstein a little, would be to see what happens when logic goes on holiday.

ACKNOWLEDGEMENTS

This paper was written while the author was holder of an Australian Bicentennial Fellowship at the Centre for Applied Philosophy and Public Ethics, University of Melbourne. The author thanks Mark Sheehan, Michael Parker, Rony Duncan, Tuija Takala, and, especially, Leslie Cannold for comments and discussion of the arguments of this paper.

NOTES

1. Matti Häyry, "A Rational Cure for Prereproductive Stress Syndrome," *Journal of Medical Ethics*, 3 (2004), p. 377.

2. *Ibid.*, p. 377.

3. Matti Häyry, "The Rational Cure for Prereproductive Stress Syndrome Revisited," *Journal of Medical Ethics*, 31 (2005), pp. 606–607.

4. Matti Häyry, *Playing God: Essays on Bioethics* (Helsinki: Helsinki University Press, 2001), chapter 3.

5. *Ibid.*, p. 32.

6. *Ibid.*, p. 40.

7. See also S. Aksoy, "Response to: A Rational Cure for Pre-reproductive Stress Syndrome," *Journal of Medical Ethics*, 30 (2004), pp. 382–383; Rebecca Bennett, "Human Reproduction: Irrational But in Most Cases Morally Defensible," *Journal of Medical Ethics*, 30 (2004), pp. 379–380; Søren Holm, "Why It Is Not Strongly Irrational to Have Children," *Journal of Medical Ethics*, 30 (2004), p. 381.

8. Häyry, "A Rational Cure for Prereproductive Stress Syndrome," p. 377.

9. Julian Savulescu, "Procreative Beneficence: Why We Should Select the Best Children," *Bioethics* 15 (2001), pp. 413–416.

10. J. Broome, *Weighing Lives* (Oxford: Oxford University Press, 2004).

11. Matti Häyry, *Liberal Utilitarianism and Applied Ethics* (London: Routledge, 1994), pp. 66–67.

12. *Ibid.*, p. 123.

13. *Ibid.*, pp. 123–124.

14. Häyry, *Playing God: Essays on Bioethics*, p. 78; See also *ibid.*, 71–72; *cf.* John Harris, *Wonderwoman and Superman: The Ethics of Human Biotechnology* (Oxford: Oxford University Press, 1993).

15. Häyry, *Liberal Utilitarianism and Applied Ethics*, p. 124.

16. Häyry, "A Rational Cure for Prereproductive Stress Syndrome," p. 377.

17. Holm, "Why It Is Not Strongly Irrational to Have Children," p. 381.

18. Aksoy, "Response to: A Rational Cure for Pre-reproductive Stress Syndrome," pp. 382-383; Bennett, "Human Reproduction: Irrational But in Most Cases Morally Defensible," pp. 379–380.

19. John Harris and Søren Holm, "Extending Human Lifespan and the Precautionary Paradox," *Journal of Medicine and Philosophy*, 27 (2002), pp. 355–368.

20. Häyry, "The Rational Cure for Prereproductive Stress Syndrome Revisited."

21. *Ibid.*, Häyry, "A Rational Cure for Prereproductive Stress Syndrome"; Matti Häyry, "If You Must Make Babies, Then At Least Make the Best Babies You Can?" *Human Fertility*, 7 (2004), pp. 105–112.

22. F. Jackson, "Decision-Theoretic Consequentialism and the Nearest and Dearest Objection," *Ethics*, 101 (1991), pp. 461–482; E. Stein, *Without Good Reason: The Rationality Debate in Philosophy and Cognitive Science* (Oxford: Oxford University Press, 1996).

23. Häyry, "The Rational Cure for Prereproductive Stress Syndrome Revisited."

24. T. L. S. Sprigge, *The Rational Foundations of Ethics* (London: Routledge, 1987).

25. Cabaret Voltaire (1986) *The Crackdown*, All tracks composed by R Kirk and S Mallinder (Virgin Records, catalogue number CVCD1, 1986), track 7.

26. Onora O'Neill, "Modern Moral Philosophy and the Problem of Relevant Descriptions," *Modern Moral Philosophy*, ed. A. O'Hear (Cambridge: Cambridge University Press, 2004), pp. 301–316.

27. S. Smilansky, "Is There a Moral Obligation to Have Children," *Journal of Applied Philosophy*, 12 (1995), pp. 41-53; Häyry, "If You Must Make Babies, Then At Least Make the Best Babies You Can?"; L. Cannold, "Do We Need a Normative Account of the Decision to Parent?" *International Journal of Applied Philosophy*, 12:20 (2003), pp. 277–290; L. Cannold, *What, No Baby? Why Women are Losing the Freedom to Mother, and How They Can Get It Back* (Fremantle, WA: Curtin University Books, 2005).

28. Richard E. Ashcroft, "Hanging Around with Jackson: Consistency in Ethical Argument and How to Avoid It," *A Life of Value: Essays for John Harris*, eds. S. Holm, M. Häyry and T. Takala (Amsterdam and New York: Rodopi, in press).

29. Broome, *Weighing Lives*, p. 37.

30. J. Broome, "Reason and motivation," *Aristotelian Society Supplementary Volume* LXXI (1997), pp. 131–146; J. Broome, "Reasons," *Reason and Value: Themes from the Moral Philosophy of Joseph Raz,* eds. R. J. Wallace, P. Pettit, S. Scheffler, and M. Smith (Oxford: Oxford University Press, 2004), pp. 28–55.

Nineteen

HUMAN REPRODUCTION: SELFISH AND IRRATIONAL BUT NOT IMMORAL

Rebecca Bennett

1. Introduction

Matti Häyry argues that not only is the choice to have children always an irrational choice but it is necessarily an immoral choice. Thus, for Häyry "human reproduction is fundamentally immoral."[1]

In this chapter I consider the arguments put forward by Häyry in order to assess his claim that it is always wrong to reproduce. I will argue that even though the choice to bring to birth a child is, on many levels, a highly irrational and an invariably selfish choice this does not necessarily make our choices to reproduce morally unacceptable. In fact I will argue that if we create a world governed by the principles Häyry advocates, not only would we fail in his aim to produce a world morally superior to our current world, but we would also produce an inferior grey and joyless world where individual autonomy is completely disregarded.

2. Häyry's Position

Häyry argues that the reason that it is irrational and immoral to choose to bring to birth a child is that "having a child can always realistically lead to the worse possible outcome, when the alternative is not having a child."[2] Häyry argues that when people consider having children they are faced with a choice between deciding not to have children and thus harming or benefitting no-one (this, it is argued has a value of zero), or choosing to have children where this life may be good or bad and thus the value of this choice can be negative, positive or zero[3]. Thus, Häyry argues, the only rational and moral course of action is to avoid suffering where possible and thus to avoid reproduction as all reproduction involves a risk of suffering.

I wish to consider this argument in three stages. Firstly, I want to explore the notion of whether existence can be seen as a good thing. Secondly, I will consider whether it is irrational to reproduce and what relevance the rationality or otherwise of this decision has on its morality. And finally I will consider whether Häyry is justified in his claim that "human reproduction is funcamen-tally immoral."[4]

3. Is it Better to Come into Existence?

There are those who argue that individuals benefit from existence and as a re-sult that we have a moral imperative to reproduce. For example, Aksoy claims that life and existence is always better than non-existence. Therefore, it is irra-tional and immoral to "sentence" someone to non-existence while you have the chance to bring them into life and existence.[5] However, such a position is logi-cally impossible to maintain.

The problem here is that no sense can be made of the claim that *someone* is sentenced to non-existence. An entity that does not exist cannot be harmed by any action or inaction. Thus, no-one exists to be harmed by not being brought to into existence. Aksoy and others who argue that being brought into existence is a benefit and non-existence a harm, argue this from the under-standable point of view that they enjoy their lives and feel they have benefited from their existence. However, as Benatar points out:

> The fact that one enjoys one's life does not make one's existence better than non-existence, because if one had not come into existence there would have been nobody to have missed the joy of leading the life and so the absence of joy would not be bad.[6]

The only sense in which existence could be a benefit is if we could identify an entity that would benefit from existence—that there were beings "in waiting" that desired existence, for instance, a religious idea of souls waiting to be em-bodied. For this unlikely scenario to have any impact on the argument, it would further need to be clear that the state of "soul in waiting" was such that existence, with its inherent suffering could be seen as a clearly preferable state. As this is completely untenable we have to accept that existence is not a mor-ally preferable state to non-existence and thus that being brought into being cannot logically be considered a benefit.

A. Selfish?

If we accept that no-one is harmed by non-existence and no-one is benefited by being brought into existence, then the desire to procreate is clearly a very self-ish desire. No sense can be made of any claims that children are created for their own sake or to improve their welfare. This claim fails for the same reason claims that existing is preferable to non-existence fail. Children are created for the sake of their parents. They are created to fulfill some desire or need that individuals have to parent a child for whatever reasons.

It is interesting that when considering certain moral dilemmas prospective parents are often called selfish when making what others deem to be unacceptable choices about reproduction. So those who wish to choose the sex of their children or any other "non-medical" trait are often condemned in this way.[7] The argument here is that the prospective parents do not want a child for its own sake but for what (they hope) it will bring to their lives. The problem with this kind of argument is, as I have already pointed out, that the creation of children is pretty much always a selfish act (with the exception perhaps of the creation of so-called "savior siblings").

B. Harmful Existence?

Not only is it impossible to be benefited from being brought into existence it is also clear that being brought into existence has the potential to be a harm. Benatar expresses the reasoning behind this effectively when he says:

> The absence of pain is good, while the absence of pleasure is not necessarily bad. This asymmetry between pain and pleasure suggests that non-existence is preferable to coming into existence. There is always some pain associated with existence, whereas non-existence involves an absence of pleasure that is not bad, because there is no existing person who is being deprived.[8]

Thus, while no-one is harmed by the lack of pleasure caused by non-existence, it is clear that individuals are caused harm by the pain inherent in existence. Thus, there can be no moral imperative to reproduce. That is, we have no duty to reproduce as we do no harm to anyone by not reproducing and we may cause harm by bringing individuals into existence.

However, although I agree with Häyry that there is no moral imperative to reproduce, Häyry mistakenly takes this conclusion one step further. He claims that as being brought into existence is not a benefit (and entails suffering) that any choice to create a new life is *necessarily* immoral. I will show later why Häyry is wrong about this further conclusion but before I explore this fundamental issue I wish to investigate the claim that the choice to reproduce is irrational and what relevance the rationality or otherwise of this decision has on its morality.

C. Irrational?

Häyry explains that:

> I believe it would be irrational to choose the course of action that can re-
> alistically lead to the worst possible outcome. And I believe that having a
> child can always realistically lead to the worst possible outcome, when
> the alternative is not to have a child.[9]

There are two main problems with Häyry's position on the irrationality of procreation. Firstly, it is not clear that choosing to have a child is *likely* to lead to
the "worst possible outcome." I will explain this later when considering more
generally the immorality of procreation. Secondly, the irrationality of choices
to procreate is important when it comes to the morality of reproduction but not
for the reasons Häyry puts forward.

As we have seen Häyry argues that the irrationality of choices to reproduce arise from the fact that these choices may "lead to the worst possible outcome."[10] However, this claim seems to have little to do with irrationality but is
more to do with the immorality of this choice. It may be foolish or irrational to
make a choice that may lead to the worst outcome but it is not the irrationality
of this choice that makes such a choice morally unacceptable. What makes the
choice morally unacceptable is if it is likely to lead to the worse possible outcome.

Indeed Häyry accepts that the irrationality of a choice does not make that
choice immoral by saying: "My moral objections to having children are not
necessarily linked with my views on the irrationality of the practice. I do not
claim human reproduction is wrong, *because* it is irrational."[11] As Häyry
agrees that the irrationality of a decision to reproduce is not what makes this
decision immoral then it seems difficult to understand why the irrationality of
human reproduction is such an issue for him. It is difficult to see why focusing
on the issue of irrationality rather than leaving it aside and merely talking
about the immorality of reproduction is anything but distracting and confusing.

However, there is a different sense in which the irrationality of choices to
reproduce is relevant to the morality of this issue. This sense is alluded to in
Häyry's work but never addressed directly. He argues that:

> Possible parents could be told that, according to at least one philosopher,
> it would be all right for them not to reproduce at all. In a social environ-
> ment where the pressure to procreate makes the choice in the majority of
> cases less than fully autonomous, this could empower people to make the
> unpopular, but if my arguments are sound, rational choice, to remain
> childless.[12]

It is the "less than fully autonomous" nature of the choice to reproduce that is important here and that deserves exploration.

For most people planning to conceive and bring to birth children, this choice is necessarily an irrational one on many levels. In most cases we choose to bring to birth children based on unquantifiable and unpredictable ideas of what they will bring to our lives and the lives of those around us. Even if we choose to bring to birth children for more pragmatic reasons such as producing children to continue the family business or provide for one's old age, it is impossible to determine whether this goal will or is even likely to be achieved. Interestingly, one of the most "rational" and perhaps one of the only unselfish reasons that might be given to make a decision to bring to birth a child is one that has created great controversy. The aim of producing a "savior child" using pre-implantation diagnosis and *in vitro* fertilization techniques to be a compatible donor for an existing ill child, would seem to be one of very few cases where the choice to create a new child could be viewed as a rational choice. However, most of us create children either for no reason at all or in an attempt to produce outcomes that can in no way be predicted or guaranteed.

I would go further and argue that not only is human reproduction irrational on many levels but as a result the choice to reproduce in many cases could not be deemed the authentic autonomous choice of the individual. To be an autonomous or authentic choice to reproduce, this choice should be based on appropriate and accurate information and not be influenced or coerced in any way. As I have already discussed choices to reproduce are mostly based on unquantifiable notions of what our child will be like and what parenting this child will bring to our lives. Further, the desire to reproduce is influenced not only by our biological and genetic make up but also by social conditioning. As a result choices to reproduce are invariably not the sort of choices that would stand up to scrutiny in terms of gauging their authenticity.

The reason why irrationality, in the sense of diminished autonomy, is important here is not because choices that are irrational or far from fully autonomous are necessarily immoral choices. We invariably act in ways that are irrational and far from autonomous. In fact many of what are considered to be the most valuable experiences in life e.g. love, sex, dancing, creating children, art, recreational drug/alcohol use, etc. may have little or no rational justification (especially based on Häyry's interpretation of rational) but their irrationality or the diminished autonomy they arise from does not render these activities necessarily immoral. The irrationality or non-autonomous nature of these choices is irrelevant to their immorality. What makes an action immoral is reliant on other factors such as whether this action harms another.

However, while irrationality and diminished autonomy do not equate to immorality, the authenticity of a decision is clearly morally relevant. It is generally accepted that respecting individual autonomy is a fundamental moral principle that enables individuals to have control over their own lives. If we accept this principle then we should not only do all we can to respect the choices of individuals but also to enable these decisions to be as fully autonomous as possible. By this we mean that what we wish to enable the individual to make is the best choice for himself based on relevant and accurate information and without pressure or coercion.

Thus, if it is clear that choices to reproduce are "less than fully autonomous" then we should do everything possible to increase the autonomy of these choices. Here I agree with Häyry that we should make sure the message goes out that "it would be all right for [people] not to reproduce at all"[13] in order to attempt to counter the social pressure to reproduce and attempt to maximize the autonomy of those considering whether to reproduce by making it clear that a decision not to reproduce is wholly acceptable on every level. This is an important notion to stress as although we might take it for granted that no-one should be made to choose to reproduce when they do not wish to, as the general assumption is that people value child rearing, then pressure is inevitably put on people in this way. It would be no bad thing to counsel individuals both for and against reproduction to allow them to make the choice that is the right one for them and their circumstances. However, if part of this counseling involves convincing individuals that reproducing is immoral this would not only, in my view, be unacceptable practically, but also theoretically and thus morally.

4. Selfish, Irrational But Immoral?

Let's recap on the argument so far. At this point (apart from this minor detail of the relevance of irrationality to immorality) it certainly may seem that Häyry is on a winning streak. I have accepted that there is no moral imperative to reproduce as all choices to reproduce (bar perhaps "savior siblings") are selfish as children are not born for their own sake. This fact is clear as it is logically impossible to make a case for the idea that existence is a morally preferable state to non-existence. I have also accepted that the choice to reproduce is irrational on many levels to the extent that it is difficult to be sure of the authenticity of this choice. Therefore, if we choose to reproduce we a) do not benefit the resultant child, b) have probably been coerced into this decision on some level by our biology and society and c) are not likely to produce the outcome we imagined when we were making our choice to reproduce as how it will feel to be a parent and what our child will become cannot be foreseen. From this it is clear that it should be made clear to people that *not* having children is a viable and completely acceptable option.

However, what of those who even after being presented with these conclusions still wish to reproduce? While their reasons for wanting to procreate are likely to be irrational on many levels and influenced by social and biological conditioning, these desires are often among the most strongly held desires people ever have. I will argue that to deny the expression of these reproductive choices, is, at least in most cases, cruel and unjustified.

5. Is Human Reproduction Fundamentally Immoral?

As we know Häyry makes a bold claim that "human reproduction is fundamentally immoral."[14] However, his justification for this claim is less clearly spelt out. He claims he has "two different objections to human reproduction."[15] The first justification is that "[s]ince all human beings suffer at some point in their lives, every parent who could have declined to procreate is to blame."[16] This is the idea that as all human existence involves suffering human reproduction is bad because it creates more people who will necessarily suffer. The second justification is based on the slightly different idea of risk avoidance. Häyry explains this notion saying "since potential parents cannot guarantee that the lives of their children will be better than non-existence, they can also be rightfully accused of gambling on other people's lives, whatever the outcome."[17] Here his argument is that human reproduction is bad because some people have bad lives, therefore we should avoid reproducing in order to avoid the risk of creating these bad lives.

These are two quite different justifications for Häyry's conclusions and it's helpful to examine them in turn.

A. Existence = Suffering = Bad

That all human beings suffer is a fact. Even those of us who feel our lives are a huge blessing and value our existence enormously suffer at some point. We all endure physical and emotional pain to some degree. Here Häyry appears to be arguing that a life that contains *any* suffering is a life that should not have been created, that is, it is an unworthwhile life, a life of negative value. Thus, the argument is that because of the suffering inherent in existence it is always a moral wrong to create new lives.

If Häyry was convinced of the strength of this argument he would be committed to the conclusion that as all lives are unworthwhile lives, not only is reproduction immoral but also that all continued human existence is immoral. If all human lives are of negative value and unworthwhile then non-existence is a clear benefit and surely the only right thing to do is to end all human existence as soon as possible. If Häyry really believes that the morally preferable course of action is that which avoids suffering where this is possible then it seems that, based on his analysis, he should be encouraging not only the avoidance of human reproduction but the ending of existing human lives including his own.

It may well be that Häyry accepts this aspect of his argument and agrees that the world would be a better place if all humans ceased to exist. This, of course, would be the eventual outcome of a world with no reproduction. He might, however, argue that to kill existing people against their will would be wrong, not because they would not be better off dead but because if they wish (irrationally and erroneously on Häyry's view) to continue to live then to kill them against their will would be a greater wrong than to remove the suffering of existence.

However, perhaps a more fundamental problem with this argument is that the notion that all lives are unworthwhile as they involve unnecessary suffering seems to contradict Häyry's argument that "the life of an individual can be good or bad" or of positive or negative value.[18] Here in one breath he argues that as all lives involve suffering they should not be created, implying a negative value to all existence, and in another breath he argues that lives can have a positive value. It seems difficult to reconcile these two claims and it seems difficult to reconcile a claim that all lives are unworthwhile with the realty of how we experience the world.

While it is easy to see how creating a child who is likely to experience great and overwhelming suffering is not only an irrational, selfish but also a morally reprehensible choice,[19] it is not clear that most or even very many children brought to birth will have such an existence. If the life we create is one that is considered a valuable and positive experience overall or as Benatar puts it a life "[w]here we can presume that those whom we bring into existence will not mind that we do,"[20] then it would seem that we produce a life that has not harmed anyone. Häyry seems to agree with this by acknowledging that life can have a positive value.

Thus, while no-one is benefited by being brought into existence, if that existence turns out to be one of positive value overall, a life that the person living it does not wish to end, then we have not done any wrong. As we have seen Häyry argues that when people consider having children they are faced with a choice between deciding not to have children and thus harming or befitting no-one (this, it is argued has a value of zero), or choosing to have children where this life may be good or bad and thus the value of this choice can be negative, positive or zero.[21] It seems that if we create lives that have a neutral, or positive value we have done no wrong, the only wrong involved in reproduction is to create lives of negative value.

The problem with this position is a practical one. While it may be morally acceptable to create lives that do not have a negative value the problem here is how we ensure that these lives are not created. It seems impossible to identify which lives will have a negative value and how we would quantify this in advance. At one end of the spectrum it will be possible to identify some rare and serious conditions that are extremely likely to render life a harm, but in most cases whether a life has negative or positive value will depend on a multitude of factors that cannot be quantified or predicted.

B. Avoiding the Risk of "Bad" Lives

This leads us to Häyry's second justification. Here he overturns his earlier justification and accepts that some lives, even though they contain suffering, may have a positive value but claims that the risk of creating a life of negative value renders any choice to reproduce immoral. The argument here is based on what Häyry calls the "maximin strategy."[22] He explains this strategy saying that when we "do not know with any certainty what the outcomes of our action or inaction will be" then "[r]easonable precaution dictates that we should not pick out policies, or courses of action, which can realistically have disastrous consequences."[23] The argument is then that if reproduction *can* produce lives that are so dominated by suffering that they have an overall negative value and we cannot eliminate the risk of this happening then reproduction should be avoided. In Häyry's first argument all lives are deemed unworthwhile because all existence creates unnecessary suffering. On this second view the only unworthwhile lives are those lives that have a negative value, lives that are not valued by those who lead them because of the overwhelming suffering these lives contain. Thus on this second view, the point here is not that reproduction *necessarily* causes suffering as some lives may well be of positive value, but that there is always the risk that reproduction will lead to the creation of lives of negative value. On this view reproduction should be avoided to avoid the risk of producing such unworthwhile and negative lives.

While these two possible justifications for Häyry's conclusion that human reproduction is fundamentally immoral are quite different in their detail and incompatible with each other they do appear to lead to the same conclusion. This conclusion is the conclusion that as reproduction unavoidably creates unnecessary suffering (either to all those who exist or to a small minority of those who exist depending on the argument taken), then we have good moral reasons to refrain from reproducing.

6. The Bigger Picture

However, while it may be true that no-one is harmed by non-existence and some are harmed by existence Häyry is wrong to assume that this leads to the conclusion that "human reproduction is fundamentally immoral."[24] The reason for erroneous conclusion is that it fails to see the bigger picture. It is true that we would avoid the suffering of newly created people if we did not create those people but what of the suffering created by repressing desires to reproduce? And further what of the consequences to the rest of human life if we apply Häyry's maximin strategy more widely?

While our desires to reproduce and rear children are invariably selfish and based on dubious reasoning these desires are incredibly strong and, for many, absolutely central goals in our lives. If we have any doubt of this consider the lengths people will go to attempt to have children: enduring risky, unpleasant, stressful (and often expensive) fertility treatment or, more commonly, enduring pregnancy, childbirth and the emotional, practical and financial burdens of being a parent. Clearly we should not impose these burdens on those who do not desire them and all efforts should be made to ensure this does not happen, however, to persuade those who do have these very strongly held desires to forgo them will cause enormous grief for a huge proportion of the population.

In response to this Häyry would argue that while he is convinced on the immorality of reproduction he does "not advocate direct counselling."[25] He argues that there is little point in reproaching individuals who are planning to have children as "the prospect of suffering will probably not deter them"[26] and thus, he argues, "the best strategy is to tolerate their immorality."[27] He seems to be arguing that while reproduction is fundamentally wrong we should not try and persuade people against reproducing. This stance is problematic on two levels. Firstly, Häyry does not seem consistent in his "live and let live" attitude. While rejecting directive counseling he does suggest that the irrationality and immorality of having children should become a legitimate part of guidance given to those expressing a wish to have children.[28] It seems difficult to see how informing prospective parents of the immorality of reproduction is non-directive counseling that allows a completely free choice.

The second problem with Häyry position here is that if he really believes that it is fundamentally morally wrong to reproduce then why would it be wrong to reproach those planning to do so? If something is morally wrong then surely it is our duty to try and prevent this moral wrong occurring?

At very least the logical conclusion to Häyry's argument is that we should try and persuade/encourage people not to reproduce and perhaps even take steps to prevent them from doing so wherever possible. Certainly, on Häyry's view, fertility treatment should be withheld from all but a small handful of cases (cases where fertility treatment was used by the fertile in order to prevent the birth of children with genetic disorders, rather than by the fertile to create new lives that otherwise would not have been created).

Further, if we accept Häyry's maximin strategy that "we should not pick out policies, or courses of action, which can realistically have disastrous consequences."[29] not only should we avoid reproducing but we should avoid all sorts of activities that, are hugely important to many of our lives. For instance, what justification do we have for having any close personal relationships let alone sexual or romantic relationships? These relationships always cause suffering even if it is only the suffering of minor arguments or bereavement but more often relationships are characterized by disastrous consequences caused by betrayal and rejection. Based on Häyry's reasoning it would seem to be not only wholly irrational, but more importantly *immoral,* to enter into such relationships as this will cause unnecessary suffering that could be avoided by avoiding these collaborations. In reply to this he might argue that the suffering caused by avoiding close relationships would be such that while avoiding such relationships might be morally preferable it would not be morally wrong to do otherwise as suffering is caused by either action. However, this is equally applicable to reproduction. If we deny ourselves the expression of our deeply held desires to reproduce this will cause a huge amount of suffering to a huge number of individuals. Perhaps desires to reproduce or enter into close relationships are not rational desires due to the unnecessary suffering these choices create and perhaps we might do better not to have these desires but as the human psyche does not work that way where does this leave us?

7. Häyry's World versus Bennett's World

Faced with this problem we seem to have two very different options open to us:

A. Häyry's World

We could attempt to create a world along the lines that Häyry's analysis suggests we should. In this world we would be encouraged to refrain from any behaviour that might have disastrous consequences and cause unnecessary suffering. Thus, in this world reproduction would be discouraged as would any kind of close relationships, dangerous sports, potentially harmful social activities (e.g. casual sex, alcohol use) etc.

B. Bennett's World

Or we could create a world where human desires such as the desire to procreate, have close relationships, etc. are supported but with the proviso that we should attempt to prevent these desires causing serious harm to others. In the realm of human reproduction this would mean discouraging individuals from creating lives that are likely to be so dominated by suffering as to render them unworthwhile. While it would be possible to counsel those thinking of reproducing and even offering screening in order to help prevent the creation of lives of negative value, it will be impossible to remove the risk of creating these lives completely.

8. Conclusions

Häyry's point in all this was to try to determine the morality of reproduction. In doing so he makes a case for the moral superiority of a world where unnecessary suffering is avoided by refraining from reproducing. But which of these two worlds described above (if either) is actually morally superior? In which world is suffering avoided? Both worlds still cannot avoid the creation of unnecessary suffering. In Bennett's world this takes the form of the unavoidable creation of some lives of negative value and other forms of suffering inherent in human activities and relationships. In Häyry's world the suffering created takes the form of the frustration or condemnation of individual's deeply held desires for procreation, close relations and other potentially dangerous practices. However, while both worlds may still contain unnecessary suffering it seems that if we consider human autonomy as important then Bennett's world has the moral edge. While Bennett's world is flawed, respect for individual autonomy is at the centre of its morality, encouraging individuals to follow their desires. In Häyry's world it seems that concern for the removal of suffering is not only unsuccessful, in that one kind of suffering is replaced by another, but also it is placed high above any concern for respecting individual autonomy. In this world individuals are encouraged not to follow their desires regarding what they wish to do with their lives even though this oppressive regime will not achieve its aim of reducing suffering.

In conclusion, while it may well be immoral to choose to bring to birth a child that is likely to have a life of negative value, this does not make human reproduction *necessarily* immoral. While we have no moral imperative to reproduce, those who wish to do so do no wrong if they take reasonable steps to attempt to ensure that any resulting child will have a life that they will value. The fact that choices to reproduce are irrational on many levels is largely irrelevant to the morality of the issue. However, what does seem to be both a rationally and morally compelling prescription is to allow individuals to make choices that, while running the small risk of creating a life of negative value, are very likely to increase the personal fulfillment and sense of autonomy of those who make them.

NOTES

1. Matti Häyry, "A Rational Cure for Prereproductive Stress Syndrome," *Journal of Medical Ethics*, 30 (2004) p. 377.

2. *Ibid.*

3. *Ibid.*

4. *Ibid.*

5. S. Aksoy, "Response to: A Rational Cure for Pre-Reproductive Stress Syndrome," *Journal of Medical Ethics*, 30 (2004), p. 383.

6. David Benatar, "Why It Is Better Never to Come into Existence," *American Philosophical Quarterly*, 34:3 (July 1997), pp. 345–355.

7. Human Fertilisation and Embryology Authority, "Sex Selection: Options for Regulation. A Report on the HFEA's 2002–03 Review of Sex Selection Including a Discussion of Legislative and Regulative Options," (London: HFEA, 2003), para 139. p. 34.

8. Benatar, "Why It Is Better Never to Come into Existence," p. 345.

9. Häyry, "A Rational Cure for Prereproductive Stress Syndrome," p. 377.

10. *Ibid.*

11. *Ibid.*, p. 378.

12. *Ibid.*

13. *Ibid.*

14. *Ibid.*, p. 377.

15. *Ibid.*, p. 378.

16. *Ibid.*

17. *Ibid.*

18. *Ibid.*, p. 377.

19. See, *e.g.*, Rebecca Bennett and John Harris, "Are There Lives Not Worth Living? When Is It Morally Wrong to Reproduce?" *Ethical Issues in Maternal-Fetal Medicine*, ed. Donna Dickenson, (Cambridge: Cambridge University Press, 2002), pp. 321–334.

20. Benatar, "Why It Is Better Never to Come into Existence," p. 345–355.

21. Häyry, "A Rational Cure for Prereproductive Stress Syndrome," p. 377.

22. *Ibid.*

23. *Ibid.*

24. *Ibid.*

25. Matti Häyry, "The Rational Cure for Prereproductive Stress Syndrome Revisited," *Journal of Medical Ethics*, 31 (2005), p. 606.

26. Häyry, "A Rational Cure for Prereproductive Stress Syndrome," p. 378.

27. *Ibid.*

28. *Ibid.*

29. *Ibid.*, p. 377.

Twenty

GAMBLING, RISKS, AND REPRODUCTION: A REPLY TO MATTI HÄYRY

Tom Buller

1. Reproductive Rights and Wrongs

People decide to have children for a variety of reasons. One might decide to do so in order to carry on the noble family line, or to have someone to look after one when one has become elderly, or to have a sibling for existent children, or because one believes that children bring joy to the world, or because one doesn't like the couple in the apartment below. Contrariwise, there are also good reasons not to have children, for example one might decide not to have children (or any more of them) because one cannot afford to do so, or because one believes that the planet is already overpopulated.

In broad terms, competent adults have the right to reproduce and this right is a negative right, a right of non-interference. In this regard, the freedom to have children is similar to the freedom to choose one's own religion, partner, or the method by which to educate one's children, for the right to reproduce serves to protect individual values and interests against the interests of others or social utility. Thus although we might all believe that the decision by Smith and Jones to have a sixth child is very poor one, indeed, given the fact that neither of them is employed, and even an irrational one given their own concerns about over-population, if there is a right to reproduce then we would not be justified in attempting to restrict their actions on purely utilitarian or paternalistic grounds.

However, the right to reproduce carries with it certain moral responsibilities and we expect prospective parents to act in a way that can be reasonably expected to benefit the future child. For example, we expect parents to participate in appropriate prenatal care and to avoid behaviors that will predictably lead to birth defects. Our social policy in this matter extends to mandating (and sometimes providing for) maternity leave, offering free prenatal care, issuing warnings about alcohol consumption and tobacco use by pregnant women,[1] and more controversial legal attempts to enforce "good behavior" among low-income pregnant women.[2,3] As Matti Häyry says, we expect prospective parents to "make the best babies" they can but this expectation is not too demanding: prospective parents are expected to be responsible, not saintly.[4]

In some cases the responsible decision may be to refrain from having a child or to terminate the pregnancy, for example, in those cases where there is a considerable likelihood that the future child will be born with profound cognitive and physical disability. Underlying such a judgment is the belief that the life of a child, like that of an adult, is worthwhile only if it is not utterly constrained by pain and suffering; if the life is considered to be so constrained and judged not to be worthwhile then, other things being equal, the life has negative value and, hence, death would be preferable.

This quality of life notion is, of course, widespread, and we frequently appeal to this notion in our decisions to withhold or withdraw life-sustaining treatment from children and adults and, more controversially, in our decisions to assist death more directly. This quality of life notion applies equally to present and future lives: if we believe that it would be irresponsible and, perhaps, immoral to continue to provide life-sustaining treatment for an existent patient whose life has negative value then, other things being equal, it would be equally wrong to bring such a life into the world. One might object that the interests of others, for example, the family, are important or that one can never accurately predict the value of future lives, but similar objections could be raised about the value of present lives. If this is correct, then in those cases where we can reasonably expect that the future life will have negative value, the morally appropriate decision may well be to refrain from having the child or to terminate the pregnancy. Thus on this analysis if Smith and Jones are both carriers for Huntington's Chorea or Tay-Sachs disease, or if it is determined that the fetus will be profoundly disabled, then Smith and Jones would not be acting responsibly if they decided to have the child. In other words, prospective parents have a responsibility to refrain from having children if the necessary, but not sufficient, condition of a worthwhile life is not met.

2. Future Children and Future Harms

According to Matti Häyry this condition is never met and hence it is always morally wrong and irrational to have children.[5] Häyry's argument for this conclusion runs as follows. Other things being equal, a person acts rationally if after careful deliberation he or she chooses the action that leads to the best outcome, consistent with the person's beliefs and values. An appropriate and familiar example of this notion is the *maximin strategy* whereby it is rational to avoid the worst possible outcome. As far as prospective parents are concerned, the worst outcome is for the future child to have a life of negative value, hence prospective parents act rationally if they seek to avoid this outcome. If prospective parents decide to have children there is a risk that the future child will have a life of negative value (either at birth or as the result of injury later in life), whereas if they decide not to have a child there is no risk that the future child will have a life of negative value. Since the decision not to have children cannot logically be better or worse for the future child, this decision has zero value. In conclusion, if parents act rationally so as to avoid the worst outcome they should decide not to have children.

Häyry's argument can be summarized as follows:

P1. It is rational to avoid the possible negative outcome when the alternative outcome has neutral or zero value.
P2. A decision not to have children has the value of zero in terms of the potential future individuals and their lives.
P3. A decision to have children has a possible negative value
C. It is rational, therefore, to choose not to have children.

Moreover, Häyry presents the following additional considerations in support of his argument. A decision to have a child is immoral because one cannot rule out the possibility that the life of (any) future child could have negative value, and, therefore, by deciding to have a child prospective parents are gambling with the life of the future child. Furthermore, although there may be benefits to the parents, siblings or others to having a child, these benefits do not outweigh the harm of a life of negative value.

As a parallel to the decision to have children, Häyry asks us to consider whether we should pass on a box that contains either jewellery or explosives (we don't know which). If we keep the box no one will be harmed but if we pass on the box there is a chance that the recipient will be badly harmed (or become rich). In such a case Häyry concludes it would be moral to keep the box and immoral to pass it on, since this latter option excludes the possibility of injury.

3. Good Bets and Bad Risks

Is Häyry's conclusion the correct one? I believe that there are a number of considerations that suggest otherwise. Let us begin by looking at the first premise of Häyry's argument and the claim that it is rational to avoid the possible negative outcome when the alternative outcome has a neutral or zero value. If the choice facing me is between a negative outcome or a neutral outcome, then, other things being equal, it makes little sense to choose the negative one. Hence we would agree with Häyry that it would be rational to choose the neutral outcome. For example, if I know that *Angry Ferret* is running in the 3:30 at Kempton Park and will certainly fail to finish, then it would be irrational and foolhardy of me to bet £50 on the horse to win. In such a case the best possible outcome is avoidance of the worst possible outcome—the best I can do is not to lose my money.

Very few choices, however, including those facing prospective parents are restricted to a choice between a negative and a neutral outcome. In one sense in fact this is no choice at all for this type of case is more accurately described as a test of rationality rather than a rational choice. It is in this sense that there is only one option when confronted with the question, "Your money or your life?" The more plausible scenario facing prospective parents is a choice among at least three outcomes: negative, neutral and positive. For example, imagine the possibility that Smith or Jones carries the gene mutation for Fragile X syndrome. If they decide to have a child then it is possible that the future child will have Fragile X syndrome or that he or she will not, or that the prospective parents are unable to conceive (or a number of other possibilities).

If we take into account these additional alternatives it is no longer clear that it would be rational for the prospective parents to choose the neutral outcome over the negative one, for it is now possible for the parents to avoid the negative outcome by choosing the option that will lead to a positive one. Thus a more likely description of the above race is that *Angry Ferret* has a chance of winning, and the question of whether it is rational to bet on this horse will be answered by all those factors that lovers of horse-racing claim to know so much about: odds, form, rider, weather, temperament, distance etc. If *Angry Ferret* is the clear favorite, the conditions are ideal and the odds generous, it would not be irrational to bet on the horse. It might be worth a bet.

If Smith and Jones are considering whether to have a child it would, of course, be rational of them to consider the possibility that the future child might have a life of negative value. Sometimes this possibility is very high and the degree of harm or suffering for the future child so great that the best outcome that they can hope for is to avoid the negative one. In these types of cases, for example if Smith and Jones are both carriers for Huntington's or Tay-Sachs, we might well agree with Häyry that it would be rational and moral for Smith and Jones to decide not to have this child. In other cases, however, the possibility and degree of harm may be low. Perhaps Smith and Jones are young and healthy, and all indications and tests determine the fetus to be thriving and lacking the harmful gene mutation; or, further down the road, perhaps their 21 year-old offspring has just completed the London Marathon, sold a successful electronics company and retired to Monaco. It is certainly possible that tragedy could strike at any time and the life of their child could end up as having negative value, but is this possibility sufficient in and by itself to make the decision to reproduce irrational? Our answer might well be the same as that we gave in regard to betting on *Angry Ferret*—it may be worth the risk. In other words, if it is more likely that the outcome will be positive and tragedy will not strike, then the decision to have children may not be irrational.

A plausible explanation for why we might think that it may be worth the risk to have a child or to bet on a horse is that probabilities matter. When we make decisions under risk we judge a decision to be rational or irrational on the basis of goals, probability and degree of harm and benefit. In this regard, the possibility that a choice might have a negative outcome, even a catastrophic one, is not sufficient to determine that this choice is rational. Consider, for example, the parents of child with leukemia who have to decide whether to enroll the child in an experimental gene therapy trial. Let us suppose that if they decide not to participate it is predicted that the child will die within six months, whereas if they do participate there is the chance that the child will die within two months or live for another three years. What should the parents decide? If their decision is to be rational it seems clear that the parents would need to take into account the present and expected quality of life of the child, the nature of the treatment and the probabilities involved. If the probability of the child dying within six months is 90% and the chance of living for another three years is 10% then the parents may well decide not to enroll in the clinical trial, but if the odds are reversed then this may be sufficient for the parents to decide to participate.

If one frames the decision to have children in terms of a choice between facing the worst possible outcome and avoiding the worst possible outcome, between a negative and a neutral value, then it is clear that we should decide to avoid the worst possible outcome. But is this approach rational? If I am cooking soup for dinner and am worried that it might be cold by the time we sit down to eat, then one way to prevent this negative outcome is simply not to make any soup. Similarly, if I am worried by the possibility of electrocution when I change the light-bulb I could decide to always work by candlelight. In a myriad of cases like these we can avoid a negative outcome by deciding not to participate in a particular course of action, and in the same vein prospective parents can avoid creating a life of negative value by deciding not to have child. But this type of reasoning borders on the fallacious, specifically a false disjunction, for the choice presented is restricted to that between inaction or catastrophe, between no supper or cold soup. But in each of these cases catastrophe can be avoided by an outcome that is not merely neutral but positive—I could keep the soup warm or be careful when changing the light-bulb.

4. Wrongful Life

I wish now to turn to the second premise of Häyry's argument and the claim that a decision not to have children has the value of zero in terms of the potential future individuals and their lives. If one accepts the claim that some future lives have negative value then, *prima facie*, it sounds legitimate to say that it would better for the child not to be born; nevertheless, I think that this way of speaking confuses the matter. A decision to have a future child determines whether or not a child will exist at all. If the decision is made not to have a child then one cannot claim that this decision is somehow "better" *for the future child* than the decision to have the child. For the decision to have the child or not determines whether there is a future child whose life can be subject of benefit or harm. In other words, we can only include considerations about what is better or worse for the child once there is child.

Häyry makes the following claim with regard to the decision to have a child, "The value of this choice, in terms of potential future individuals and their lives, is zero." [6] In one sense this is logically true: if one decides not to have children, then there is no future child. Hence this decision has no value for the non-existent future child. Nevertheless, Häyry's conclusion that reproduction is irrational and immoral rests on a comparison between a wrongful life of negative value and this non-existent future life of zero value, and this comparison is made implicitly in terms of harms to the future child. (If this is not the case and the comparison is in terms of some other factor, what is it?) In other words, despite the fact that a future life cannot logically have value it is seen as superior in comparison to a wrongful life.

5. Gambling and Children

Should we gamble on our children's lives? It is impossible to avoid doing so. We gamble on our children's lives every time we feed them, bath them or send them to school. No matter what we do we can neither guarantee their safety nor secure their futures, and every carefully planned and well-intentioned action could end in disappointment or disaster. But although having children is a gamble it is not a lottery—care and attention do better than indifference and recklessness. It is a good idea to wear your seat belt, to keep the kids out of the kitchen, to ban firearms, and to inoculate children. In other words, we can shorten the odds in our children's favor.

In addition, the potential benefits to others can be substantial. A particular example of this is the case of Molly Nash. Molly was born with Fanconi anemia an often fatal disease in which the body fails to manufacture blood cells normally. Molly's best chance of survival was a stem cell transplant with matched cells. Through pre-implantation genetic diagnosis Molly's parents selected an embryo that was free from Fanconi anemia. Once the child, Adam, was born, cells were successfully transplanted from Adam's umbilical cord blood into Molly.

The Nash case has generated considerable discussion. One might have deontological reservations about using Adam Nash as a means to an end or about "designer babies," but the central question to ask is whether we think that the Nash's actions were rational and moral. It is certainly true that their decision was risky because the transplant might not have been successful. Consider, for example, the effect that the failure of the transplant would have had on Molly and Adam. Nevertheless, the decision to have the child (Adam) offered the possibility of saving Molly's life, and six years on the decision appears to have been a good one since all members of the family are doing well.

One can argue that the Nash's actions were rational in the sense that pre-implantation genetic diagnosis is predictable, increases probabilities and in this case was consistent with their goals and values. Furthermore, their actions were moral in deontological and utilitarian terms on the grounds that it could be argued that the parents were acting dutifully, and that the overall welfare was increased—there are now four happy, healthy lives when there could have been only two.

Perhaps Häyry would regard the Nash case as exceptional since in the normal course of events one child does not have the opportunity or capability to save a sibling's life in such a direct way. The problem with this response is it assumes the very point that Häyry denies, namely that we are able to predict what future harms will occur. (Recall that Häyry argues that any future life could be of negative value and hence it is irrational and immoral to have children). As genetic testing, therapy, and pre-implantation genetic diagnosis increases, one might contend that it will become more likely that future children will be able to offer such significant benefits to their older siblings. If this is correct, then perhaps it will become even more rational and moral to have children. Alternatively, Häyry might respond that such utilitarian considerations should never outweigh the possibility of a future life of negative quality. In reply, one can repeat the point that probabilities matter.

Contrary to Matti Häyry, I think that it is sometimes irrational and immoral to have children rather than always so. I agree with Häyry that any future life can have negative value and that we can prevent this happening by deciding not to have children. But I disagree with Häyry's conclusion that the decision to have children is, therefore, irrational and immoral. In those cases where it can be reasonably predicted that the life of the child will have negative value, then Häyry may be correct; but in those case where there is no basis for such a prediction, or where we believe that the life will have positive value, then the decision to have children is morally and rationally defensible.

NOTES

1. *E.g.*, section 04.21.065 of the current Alaska Statutes.

2. *E.g.*, *Ferguson v. City of Charleston*, 532 U.S. 67, 72 (2001).

3. Alexander Capron, "Punishing Mothers," *Hastings Center Report*, 28:1 (1998), pp. 31–34.

4. Allen Buchanan et al., *"From Chance to Choice: Genetics and Justice,"* (Cambridge: Cambridge University Press, 2000), pp. 156–159.

5. Matti Häyry, "If You Must Make Babies, Then At Least Make the Best Babies You Can?" *Human Fertility*, 7:2 (2004), pp. 105–112, and Matti Häyry, "A Rational Cure for Prereproductive Stress Syndrome," *Journal of Medical Ethics*, 30 (2004), pp. 377–378.

6. Häyry, "A Rational Cure for Prereproductive Stress Syndrome," p. 377.

Part Six

PHILOSOPHICAL RESPONSES
TO ENHANCEMENTS

Twenty-One

DO WE HAVE AN OBLIGATION
TO MAKE SMARTER BABIES?

Lisa Bortolotti

1. Introduction

In this chapter I consider some issues concerning cognitive enhancements and
the ethics of enhancing in reproduction and parenting. I argue that there are
moral reasons to enhance the cognitive capacities of the children one has, or of
the children one is going to have, and that these enhancements should not be
seen as an alternative to pursuing important changes in society that might also
improve one's own and one's children's life. It has been argued that an emphasis on enhancing cognitive capacities might encourage the commodification of
children. But this objection seems misplaced. The reasons why one decides to
reproduce can be subject to moral approbation or condemnation, as such reasons might be indicators of the quality of one's parenting and the happiness of
the future persons one is committed to bringing to life. However, once the decision to reproduce is made, no further harm comes from taking as few risks as
possible on behalf of the persons to whom one is giving life with their health,
character and cognitive capacities.

In his 2004 paper "If you must make babies, then at least make the best
babies you can?" Matti Häyry (2004)[1] defends three claims: (1) that to have
children is not necessarily good or rational; (2) that it would be good and rational to make sure that the children we do have have the best possible lives;
(3) that it is not easy to judge whether scientific advances (e.g. the possibility
of embryo selection by IVF) or social changes are the best means to achieve
this outcome. On the basis of a harmed-condition account of disability, I shall
challenge the assumption, implicit in (3), that conferring benefits by enhancements and by social change are mutually exclusive. Then I shall argue in favor
of (2) and dismiss some common objections to cognitive enhancements
(safety, allocation of resources and diminished agency). I shall also discuss the
view according to which the adoption of enhancing strategies in reproduction
and parenting is an instance of a general tendency towards the commodification of children. In working out what commodification entails, I shall argue in
favor of (1), but from a different perspective from Häyry's. I shall claim that

the motivation people have to reproduce might be more or less morally acceptable, but once the decision to reproduce is made, no further harm can come
from enhancing the (future) child's capacities.

2. Moral Reasons for Enhancing

In this chapter I defend the view that we have moral reasons to enhance. The
basis for my defense of enhancements is the principle of beneficence, according to which people have a moral obligation to prevent harm and to confer
benefits when it is possible. But the presence of moral reasons to enhance does
not imply that people have any moral obligation to use any specific enhancement strategy in conferring benefits to their (future) children. An "enhancing
strategy" is any activity that aims at preventing harm and conferring benefit.
On this account, organizing music instruction for one's children when they are
aged 3-9 is an enhancing strategy, if it is true that there is a correlation between music instruction in young children and increased spatio-temporal and
mathematical abilities.[2]

There is a gulf between recognizing moral reasons to enhance and arguing that we should be morally obliged to adopt one specific enhancing strategy
in reproduction or parenting. And that is why the debate on enhancements cannot be exhausted by an appeal to beneficence and the harm-benefit continuum.
There are pressing questions that must be raised and answered. How powerful
are the moral reasons we have for enhancing? Are there any moral reasons
against enhancing as such? What are the risks and costs involved in enhancing? Are there any moral reasons against any specific enhancing strategies?
For instance, Häyry[3] discusses one objection to embryo selection in assisted
reproduction as enhancing strategy. The process necessary for assisted reproduction might place an unnecessary burden on women, who would be required
to go through extensive testing and potentially distressful or painful procedures. All these considerations must be taken into account in our decision-
making and only those measures that seem to have reasonable costs should be
adopted in order to enhance.

A. Disability

In the so-called *harmed condition* account of disability, conditions are regarded as disabling if they are physical or mental conditions that are harmful to
the individual. According to this account, disabling conditions constitute a disadvantage with respect to relevant alternatives, not necessarily with respect to
the conditions of the typical human. The reason why the notion of normal species functioning is unhelpful in defining disabilities is that it would make disability too narrow. Changing environmental factors, or new discoveries about
the onset of serious diseases, for instance, might make it the case that typical

conditions of our species come to be regarded as disabling. Attention-deficit disorders, memory loss and Down's syndrome are disabling, because, to different extent, they cause harm to the people who are in them by exposing them to risks, impairing them in what they do, limiting their opportunities or preventing them from having experiences that are worthwhile.[4]

This conception of disability is sufficiently broad to cover all the harmful conditions that we might intuitively regard as disabling, whether the harm be primarily caused by medical conditions of the person, cognitive, genetic or environmental factors or social context. Moreover, it has clear advantages with respect to a merely *social* conception of disability, as it is not committed to the rather implausible claim that all disabling features of the condition would disappear if society were inclusive and free from discrimination or prejudice. Whereas it is certainly true that certain attitudes in society towards people who are perceived as different cannot but make things worse for disabled people, in many cases, perhaps most cases, their condition would remain harmful once society had been reformed (think again about attention-deficit disorders, memory loss or Down's syndrome).

What do I mean by "harm" in this context? I would like to adopt a very broad conception of harm as the set-back of interests or preferences about states of affairs that significantly affect an individual's well-being. It could harm me not to be able to appreciate a spectacular sunset on the coast, because I would have an interest in enjoying that view. It would increase the quality and richness of my experiential life. It would have harmed me to be born in 1774 rather than in 1974, because I would have had limited capacity to exercise my autonomy in a society in which women were less likely to receive an education, participate in public life and make their own choices.

The adoption of the harmed-condition account of disability has important consequences for our way of conceiving reproductive and parental choices. Once we accept that disabling conditions are harmful to the individual (by definition), it is easy to see that we have moral reasons to prevent disabling conditions if possible or reduce their harmful effects, as part of our commitment to the basic moral principle of avoiding unnecessary harm. But, again, this says nothing about the way in which these moral reasons might impact in practice on our choices. One might recognize the presence of moral reasons to prevent disabling conditions or reduce their harmful effects and still object on moral or other grounds to the methods by which the obligation can be carried out given a rational costs/benefits analysis. Moreover, the strength of the moral reasons we have to prevent disabilities might be thought to vary in accordance with the context of the disabling condition, and in accordance with the degree of harm that the disabling condition is likely to cause to (future) children. Many feel that we have a moral obligation to prevent a serious disability, but do not feel the same about a minor disability, which is going to cause just a slight inconvenience.

B. The Continuum between Harms and Benefits

If we accept that there are moral reasons to prevent or eradicate disability when possible, does this commit us to recognize that we also have moral reasons to enhance? Many have the intuition that there are moral reasons to avoid harm by preventing our children from being in disabling conditions, but view enhancements with suspicion. This intuition is an illusion for whoever is committed to the existence of the *harm-benefit continuum*. The harm-benefit continuum is the idea that "the reasons we have not to harm others or creating others who will be unnecessarily harmed are continuous with the reasons we have for conferring benefits on others if we can."[5] We seem to have moral reasons to improve the conditions in which others find themselves, whether these conditions are disabling or not. The reasons we have to avoid harming others are continuous with the reasons we have for conferring benefits on others if we can, because all actions are re-describable as omissions and vice versa.[6]

This is supported by the intuitive analogy between disability and enhancement. If disabling conditions constitute a *disadvantage* with respect to some relevant alternatives, enhanced conditions constitute an *advantage*. Let me offer an example. Research suggests that patients who suffer from sleep deprivation are at risk of developing cognitive and emotional difficulties, are slower at solving math's problems and processing language and are much more prone to accidents when driving. Some amphetamines are used to counterbalance the effects of sleep deprivation and they do so by improving attention, concentration, spatial working memory, and planning and have been long used by the US military for these purposes.[7] Drugs that are safer and non-addictive can have similar effects and could be used not to counteract the effects of a disabling condition but to improve performance, e.g. to help students perform well during examinations. It might seem uncontroversial to grant that an improved cognitive performance would constitute an advantage on the assumption that the enhancing drugs are safe, but some maintain that there are moral objections to using drugs for this purpose. Some are concerned that there is less worth in achieving an objective such as passing an examination if one relies on the effects of chemical substances on one's brain, or that unfairly distributed advantages will deeply affect an already unjust society. I am going to discuss these interesting objections to enhancements in the next section.

C. Changing Society

But before let me go back for a second to the moral justification of enhancements in reproduction and parenting. Some might feel that, although there are moral reasons to confer benefits, adopting enhancing strategies to do so is not the best available course of action, as it precludes other, less controversial, ways of doing it. For instance, Häyry[8] presents the promotion of social changes as an alternative to enhancement if one wants to improve the life of one's (future) children. But I cannot see how changing society and improving conditions in an individual would ever be mutually exclusive or even competing courses of action. If I have a child who is cognitively impaired, I might want to act on the surrounding social environment with the hope that, as a consequence, he will be better accepted by his peers and that he will receive more support from his teachers, but my commitment to changing society for the better is not incompatible with reducing the harm that the disability is causing to my child by intervening on his disabling condition. Similarly, in the case of a prenatal test revealing that my future child will have such a disability, I might want to take measures to prevent or reduce its potential effects on him and at the same time strengthen my commitment to creating a fairer world around him. In the circumstances in which the disability is so serious that parents come to believe that their future child will not have a life worth living, they might decide to terminate the pregnancy. But even in these extreme circumstances, it is not clear to me that they are confronted with a choice between changing society or changing the individual, or that they are sending any negative messages to other parents in similar circumstances who have taken a different course of action.

3. Moral Reasons Not to Enhance

A. Safety

In the bioethical literature, the press, and even in recent cinematography, enhancements are viewed with great suspicion. First, there are concerns about the safety of the procedures involved. Second, there are worries about the limited amount of knowledge even experts have about the consequences of, say, genetic engineering in cognitive domains. In Daniels (2005) we find an interesting example.[9] Suppose that we learn that an enhancement of short-term memory would benefit many of our cognitive processes and that we have the opportunity to enhance short-term memory by operating on embryos. Daniels argues that we should not do it because we would not be able to predict the consequences of enhancing memory performance. Daniels' concern is that enhancements might not really improve the quality of life. He is not just reiterating the idea that there are always risks involved in changing something that is working well enough. He is saying that, given the nature of certain modifications and the complex way in which we would need to assess their consequences, the fact that the capacity or trait to be enhanced is a necessary condition for better performance does not mean that by enhancing it we would produce an overall better offspring. Another example of this phenomenon is the study that has been conducted at the University of Pennsylvania on mice. Mice which had been genetically engineered to improve their memory and learning were then shown to be unusually sensitive to pain.[10]

Safety concerns should definitely be taken into account, and it is reasonable to assume that a careful risk/benefit analysis would not recommend many procedures that aim at enhancing complex cognitive functions at this stage. This fact, though, does not seem relevant to deeming enhancements *per se* unethical. What would be unethical is to risk people's health by enhancing their cognitive performance if the foreseen benefit is not worth the risk. Of course, separate issues are whether we can obtain non-biased information about safety, how the risk/benefit ratio should be calculated and by whom. It is a platitude that the perception of risk might vary and that some people might value the achievements made possible by enhanced conditions more than others. It is reported that many athletes would take a drug that would enable them to win every competition for a few years, even if the drug shortened their life significantly.[11]

B. Limited Resources

Safety aside, some people are worried about unfair allocation of resources. It is a common thought that some enhancing strategies such as genetic engineering are going to be very expensive and that only the better-off in society will be able to afford them. As a consequence, the current divisions in society will become even less bridgeable. Notice that this is not an ethical objection to enhancing as such, but a concern about the unfair distribution of resources. Actually, the worry about the ways in which enhancements will be distributed implies that enhancements are perceived as a good thing. The problem of resource allocation is an extremely urgent one, but it is not specific to cognitive enhancement in any interesting way. For all the available resources which can be seen as beneficial to humans (e.g. food, education, therapies etc.), there is an unfair distribution in society. If cognitive enhancements are going to be a further available resource, the problem of access would apply to them too. Mehlman suggests a way in which some fair access could be promoted:

> A better approach would be to permit cognitive enhancements to be available on the open market for those who can afford them and to subsidize access to them for those who cannot. ... By making these products widely available, society would gain the benefits of achievements they made possible and reduce or at least refrain from exacerbating the inequalities that stemmed from differences in wealth.[12]

Policy regulations and issues of state intervention in the research on cognitive enhancement and the availability of enhancing strategies will have to be thought out by paying attention to short- and long-term consequences, but these measures would not and do not amount to an objection to enhancing on the basis that enhancing is unethical.

C. Diminished Agency

Finally, some believe that the practice of enhancing and genetically engineering capacities will lead to a revision of our conception of agency.[13] Agents typically enjoy a certain amount of freedom of action and are subject to judgments of praise for their achievements and of blame for their failures. But if the physical or intellectual achievement of the agent is only marginally due to effort and discipline and mainly due to the effects of, say, a powerful drug, the achievement might no longer be a good reason to admire the agent. The argument is supposed to show that a pervasive use of enhancement might lead to a diminished sense of agency and responsibility.

To assess the force of this argument one needs to be able to account for what the consequences of the practice of enhancement would really be for our conception of agency. Partly, this is an empirical question. We know what our current psychological reactions to illicit drug-taking by athletes are; we feel it is cheating. But the scenario in which everybody is given an opportunity to enhance some of their conditions safely is significantly different and our reactions would almost certainly reflect that difference. It is not at all obvious that we would lose the sense of ownership of our own actions if the capacities that made it possible for us to achieve something desirable had been enhanced. One possible consequence of pervasive enhancement could be a "raising the bar" effect that would subtract little to the merits of the personal achievements of the individual.

That said, it seems as if the diminished agency objection is on to something. Suppose you are a runner and want to increase your speed by 20%. Also suppose that there are two methods by which you can achieve this target. You can take a pill that has an immediate enhancing effect on your speed or you can train for two months, three hours a day. Notice that these are both *enhancing* strategies if we define enhancements on the basis of their predicted outcomes. Now, you might have a morally relevant reason to prefer the hard way to the easy way. You might value self-discipline and think that you will grow as a person if you achieve this target by making a conscious effort to perfect your body during the next two months. You might believe that the sense of satisfaction you would get at the end of the training for having achieved the target is worth the time and the effort that are required. But all these considerations do not amount to judging that it would be unethical for you to choose the *easy* option.

An analogous case can present itself when we are considering the ethics of enhancing cognitive capacities or cognitive performance in the context of reproductive choices. To give a child the opportunity to learn how to play a musical instrument might be regarded as important, because receiving music instruction is a valuable experience independently of its alleged effects on memory and mathematical skills. It is valuable because it is formative, it is social and it might install certain values in the child, such as the idea that hard work pays off and that almost nothing rewarding in life comes cheap. If there was a magic pill that could produce the same enhancing effects immediately, would it be unethical to administer it to a child? The enhancing pill is not equivalent to music instruction, because taking the pill is not a formative experience, but it would not be unethical either. Moreover, some children do not get any pleasure out of studying music and would not respond positively to music instruction. For them, one could argue, taking the pill would not be a worse option. Their cognitive capacities would be enhanced to the same extent by hypothesis, and they would always have the opportunity to get the other benefits associated with music instruction from other formative and social experiences in their lives.

4. Commodification of Children

Häyry (2004) reviews the reasons why people make a conscious decision to have babies in spite of the obvious fact that the future persons they generate might suffer in the course of their lives. The assessment of the reasons for reproducing is not the main concern of this paper, but I need to address another common ethical objection to enhancing in reproduction, the so-called commodification of children, and the rationality of reproduction and commodification are importantly related issues. One of the most popular objections to enhancing one's children's cognitive capacities is that it encourages parents to conceive of their children as commodities, as objects that have a value not in themselves but as means to achieve something else. Why do people want trendier clothes, cars or mobile phones? Because their aesthetic properties reflect on the image of the person who owns them. One might argue that to want a smarter child is an instance of the same kind of behavior. Parents, actual or prospective, might regard their children as a means to achieve status, as something to boast about, and not as persons whose life is valuable in itself.

My view is that, once one makes the important decision to have children, there are moral reasons to do whatever is in one's power to make sure that one's children will have a happy life. This might include enhancing their cognitive abilities by methods that one finds acceptable given their risks and costs. Obviously, there are many things one cannot have control over and one can never have any certainty that one's children will be happy people. This is presumably why Häyry concludes that it is irrational to reproduce. But to claim that there are moral reasons to enhance is not sufficient to dismiss the commodification objection. The way in which parents conceive of their children has moral relevance and should be discussed, but not just in relation to enhancement. The commodification of children as an objection to enhancing in reproduction is misplaced, as it should be viewed as an objection to reproduction *tout court*.

It is often thought that people should not have merely "selfish" reasons to reproduce. The way they conceive of their children might be an indicator of poor parenting skills and might affect their capacity to bring about their children's happiness as well as their own. (This is an empirical claim and as such needs to be supported by evidence, but it has some initial plausibility.) We experience uneasiness when we read interviews to successful career women in their late thirties or early forties who declare that the only thing missing in their lives is a child, as if reproducing were the answer to a need for variety of experiences in one's life or another target to tick off on an imaginary list of things to achieve by a certain age. Our uneasiness does not necessarily track the presence of wrongdoing. After all, people might have equally respectable and yet different reasons to make the choice of having children and personal realization is likely to play a role in almost all the life-changing decisions we make. However, my point is that, if there is a commodification of children objection to reproduction, it is certainly not confined to the practice of enhancement. Commodification seems to be a complex phenomenon whose origin can be found in the motivations people have to reproduce and whose manifestations can vary. Refraining from enhancing would not necessarily contribute to changing such a conception of children.

5. Conclusion

In this chapter I have argued that people have moral reasons to enhance the cognitive performance of their children on the basis of the principle of beneficence and subject to an evaluation of the risks and costs of the chosen enhancing strategies. To further support my argument, I have defended three claims: (1) the practice of enhancement does not rule out the attempt to better one's children's life by changing society and in particular by eliminating prejudice against diversity; (2) the objections to enhancement that concern safety, allocation of resources and diminished agency do not seem to offer moral reasons against enhancements *per se*; (3) the common thought that enhancing might promote a view of children as commodities seems confused. The commodification of children is a social phenomenon of which enhancement can be a manifestation, but which has its roots in the morally dubious reasons people might have to reproduce and which can manifest itself in numerous other ways.

ACKNOWLEDGEMENTS

I am indebted to John Harris for a thorough discussion of the relation between disability and enhancements and to Matteo Mameli for very useful feedback on the arguments I have defended here. I also acknowledge the stimulus and support of the EURECA project in the preparation of this paper. The project EURECA on delimiting the concept of research and research activities was sponsored by the European Commission, DG-Research as part of the Science and Society research programme 6th Framework.

NOTES

1. Matti Häyry, "If You Must Make Babies, Then At Least Make the Best Babies You Can?" *Human Fertility*, 7:2 (2004), pp. 105–112.
2. Lois Hetland, "Learning to Make Music Enhances Spatial Reasoning," *Journal of Aesthetic Education*, 34 (2000), 179–238; Amy Graziano, Matthew Peterson and Gordon Shaw, "Enhanced Learning of Proportional Math Through Music Training and Spatio-Temporal Training," *Neurological Research* 21:2 (1999), 139–152.
3. Häyry, "If You Must Make Babies, Then At Least Make the Best Babies You Can?" p. 111.
4. Lisa Bortolotti and John Harris, "Disability, Enhancement and the Harm-Benefit Continuum," *Freedom and Responsibility in Reproductive Choice*, eds. J. Spencer and A. Pedain (Oxford and Oregon: Hart Publishing, 2006), pp. 31–49.
5. John Harris, "One Principle and Three Fallacies of Disability Studies," *Journal of Medical Ethics*, 27 (2001), pp. 383–387, p. 386.
6. Jonathan Glover, *Causing Death and Saving Lives* (New York: Penguin, 1977). John Harris, *Violence and Responsibility* (London: Routledge & Kegan Paul, 1980).
7. Anjan Chatterjee, "Cosmetic Neurology: The Controversy Over Enhancing Movement, Mentation and Mood," *Neurology*, 63 (2004), pp. 968–974, p. 969. Maxwell Mehlman, "Cognition-Enhancing Drugs," *The Millbank Quarterly*, 82:3 (2004), pp. 483–506, p. 484.
8. Häyry, "If You Must Make Babies, Then At Least Make the Best Babies You Can?" pp. 109–111.
9. Norman Daniels, "Can Anyone Really Be Talking About Ethically Modifying Human Nature?" *The Enhancement of Human Beings*, eds. Julian Savulescu and Nick Bostrom (Oxford: Oxford University Press, 2005).
10. Ya-Ping Tang, Eiji Shimizu et al., "Genetic Enhancement of Learning and Memory in Mice," *Nature*, 401 (1999), pp. 63–69; Ya-Ping Tang, Eiji Shimizu et al., "Do 'Smart' Mice Feel More Pain or Are They Just Better Learners?" *Nature Neuroscience*, 4:5 (2001), pp. 453–454.
11. Mehlman, "Cognition-Enhancing Drugs", p. 487.
12. *Ibid.*, p. 499.
13. Michael Sandel, What's wrong with enhancement, Council of Bioethics, http://www.bioethics.gov.background.sandelpaper.html (2002).

Twenty-Two

YOUTHFUL LOOKS
—NO MATTER WHAT IT COSTS?

Heta Aleksandra Gylling

"How sad it is!" murmured Dorian Gray with his eyes still fixed upon his own portrait. "How sad it is! I shall grow old, and horrible, and dreadful. But this picture will remain always young. It will never be older than this particular day of June .... If it were only the other way! If it were I who was to be always young, and the picture that was to grow old! For that— for that—I would give everything!" (Oscar Wilde, *The Picture of Dorian Gray*.)

1. Introduction

"Understanding is sublime, wit is beautiful. Courage is sublime and great, artfulness is little but beautiful" wrote Immanuel Kant in his *Observations on the Feeling of the Beautiful and Sublime*.[1] Even if it is considered to be nice and proper to emphasize inner beauty and nobleness of character when assessing the merits of our fellow beings, the fact remains that physical beauty or what is considered to be beautiful and attractive in a particular culture predominantly occupies our mind, especially when appraising the other sex. Prettiness, attractiveness or at least a pleasant appearance is what we want others to see in us. We want to appeal, we want to be praised—not only for our wit and intelligence, but also for how we look and compare to others.

In order to improve their lot, handed down by birth and heritage, both men and women have always been prone to spare no efforts in amending their looks. Faces have been painted, hair dyed, skin tattooed or body pierced, ear lobes and necks elongated; and only lack of imagination has put a limit to the variety of spectacular headgear and attire worn by our ancestors in the hope of heightening their charms and allure. This desire to appeal and to please has been dominant in all but the most austere conditions and therefore seems to be part of what it means to be human. Whether this empirical observation should have any normative relevance is of course another story.

The rapid advances of new technologies have affected our Western lifestyle not only by promising us a genetically engineered brighter future, but also by offering a possibility to try to satisfy human vanity. Plastic surgery has turned out to be an efficient tool in sculpting our features and figures to desired proportions and forms. The improvement of surgical techniques and various implants has enabled plastic surgery to rise from a medical branch which tried to save and cure suffering patients to a lucrative client-oriented business, marketed as unproblematically as new haircuts or artificial nails. First it cast its spell on women, but now an increasing number of men have found its promises rather tempting. Especially the rich American woman in vogue seems to be compelled to visit her plastic surgeon at regular intervals if she is not willing to relapse into an unkempt and sloppy existence which could easily cost her her job and social status. Even if excessive eagerness to maintain youthful looks is frowned upon, even ridiculed, the fact remains that the advances made in cosmetic surgery make it a tempting alternative to a growing number of people in affluent Western or Westernized societies.

2. The Boundaries of Rationality

But what lies behind this increasing urge to have oneself cut and stretched for often a heavy price? There is plenty of evidence showing that even those who seem to be satisfied with the end result seem to have suffered more than they expected. Even if the operation itself can be performed rather painlessly, the pains, the discomfort and length of the healing period have taken many by surprise. And even if the techniques have improved and knowledge about potential risks has increased, some operations still fall short of success. They may turn out badly either aesthetically or medically, causing serious and permanent health problems to their victims. Why then would anybody want to engage in these activities? Is it a reflection of lost confidence in our inner worth, a sign of twisted values somehow typical of our age and therefore something that should be strongly disapproved or morally condemned? Or is it unnatural in the sense that it would be justifiable to maintain that willingness to risk major cosmetic surgery is a sure sign of diminished rationality, which allows paternalistic interference? Or should we stoically accept the fact that our vanity needs its outlet and admit that accusing people of being irrational or imprudent may mean different things, ranging from genuine mental incompetence or disorder to mild differences of opinion.

The most elementary form of rationality usually requires that a person's beliefs and preferences form a more or less consistent whole and that she is capable of understanding the potential consequences of her actions. And even if we don't agree, we may see the logic in someone's wish to have her mouth reshaped or his pate planted with hair. But if somebody tries to argue that his life would be a thousand times better if his healthy, working legs were amputated, we might well be justified in saying that his rationality or sanity, i.e. his competence for autonomous decision-making is seriously flawed. We know that legs fulfill a function of moving which is an essential part of our idea of being human, which in itself does not mean that those confined to wheelchairs would somehow lose their human value when losing the ability to walk. A certain functionality is in our interest in the sense that cutting off a nose is not comparable to rhinoplasty. No matter what the shape of the nose, as long as it exists it is useful for sneezing. Surely it cannot be accepted that people have unlimited freedom to butt into each other's affairs whenever they see behavior they personally dislike. On the other hand, if serious harm might befall a person because he is not capable of sufficiently autonomous decision-making, then paternalism may be acceptable.

3. From Treatment to Aesthetic Enhancement

Youth and youthfulness are trendy in our culture—although not necessarily in theory. Certainly, we do hear people profess the worth of inner self and character, eagerly claiming that mature beauty that comes with age should not be shunned but instead praised in the light of life's polymorphism. Still, this eloquence, even if sincerely expressed, doesn't eliminate our fear of losing those physical features and characteristics we took for granted when young. Even Immanuel Kant, who was brought up in strict piety and is seen as an unemotional man who indulged in neither vices nor luxuries, saw female aging as a major threat, shadowing every woman's life:

> Finally age, the great destroyer of beauty, threatens all these charms; and if it proceeds according to the natural order of things, gradually the sublime and noble qualities must take the place of beautiful, in order to make a person always worthy of a greater respect as she ceases to be attractive.
>
> Nevertheless, when the epoch of growing old, so terrible to every woman, actually approaches, she still belongs to the fair sex, and that sex disfigures itself if in a kind of despair of holding this character longer, it gives way to surly and irritable mood.[2]

Should we simply accept the fact that losing our looks may lessen our market value or even our quality of life and disapprove of those who want to condemn others who are willing to try to restore their looks? In what follows I shall try to shed some light on this issue by analyzing different types of reconstructionist desires.

Even if the enthusiasm to embellish has survived with sparkling vitality, occasional religious forays have kept alive austere views warning, especially women, of the dangers of frivolity. A modest demeanor, the religious argument goes, gives a woman respectability without which she is liable to the vagaries of everyday life. Even if these extreme ideas are nowadays seldom encountered, one of the basic tenets of our Christian inheritance is a strong belief in the acceptance of the natural order of things. Soap and water don't necessarily form the upmost limits of personal beautification, but a surgeon's scalpel, on the other hand, may still signify preposterous folly. The question is why would any sensible person want to risk her health and suffer the pains of plastic surgery just in order to make herself look—supposedly, at least—more attractive?

Firstly, the reason for wishing to be operated does not always lie in poor self-image or an exaggerated fear of being pitied by others. Sometimes it is simply a question of such deformity that the only way the person can mentally survive and live something resembling an ordinary life, is to resort to massive operations. Even if the person himself accepts his lot of solitary existence, the reactions of others can pain his life. Vulgar curiosity makes people stare and embarrassment causes excessive avoidance; shunning which may hurt as much as physical violence. These cases are basically what plastic surgery was originally meant to deal with so that those who accept medical interference in traditional somatic therapy shouldn't have any difficulties in admitting the benefits of reconstructive plastic surgery.

Secondly, there are cases where a certain feature or slight deviation from what might be called normal, necessitates an operation. It could be the case that even if most of us were to notice this particular defect, it would not in the least affect our social relations with the person in question. The defect— defined as a defect by the person herself—may cause anguish and frustration. Genuine distress affects enjoying life and joining in social activities, and thus justifies a person's wish to have her looks altered—irrespective of what we might feel in a similar situation. If one has good reasons to ameliorate one's quality of life, why not do so? If without an operation the person would suffer from psychological trauma, the treatment should not be considered any different from other operations which all carry a certain risk. If, for instance, constant depression could be eliminated by fixing somebody with a new nose, wouldn't it be a better option than to pump the poor person full of anti-depressants? It may be easy to tell other people that their worries have clouded their judgment, but this of course does not mean that the speaker would be right merely because the same kind of mishap wouldn't cause her any serious distress. Respect for autonomy often demands belief in the sincerity and authenticity of others' feelings.

But how should we feel about those who apparently, without any visible reason, are ready to have their faces lifted, noses and lips reshaped, thighs liposucted or who are ready—instead of just being nipped and tucked—to add alien parts to their bodies. If rumors are to be believed, breast implants might become more the rule than the exception while some men have felt that their male ego has to be fortified with the help of some extraordinary surgical measures on their genitals.

But would it be justifiable to condemn those who subject themselves to more or less painful operations, those who are ready to risk their physical health for the allegedly greater benefits of aesthetic lure? Many seem to think that the problem somehow lies in the misuse of medicine. Plastic surgery should be left to benefit those in serious need of operation and should not be used as a plaything for those with more money than sense. But the smaller the risk in a particular operation, the more difficult it is to argue for its wrongness. The sterile nature of plastic surgery doesn't really separate it from body piercing and tattoos and thereby render it more immoral. And even if we know that massive surgical operations are not the same as applying mascara and powder or wearing a manly toupee, both belong to the realm of self-adornment and cannot really be doomed by reference to a radical violation of the laws of nature.

Among those ready to condemn cosmetic surgery many would be inclined to say that piercing women's earlobes is merely an instance of harmless self-mutilation. But why then, would the same people feel disgusted by adult body piercing? The main answer of course lies in our tendency to feel disgusted by things unfamiliar to us, at least in the sense that we could not imagine something for ourselves. Our reactions towards body piercing may vary from silent acceptance in the name of individual autonomy (I myself belonging to that category), to either serious moral disgust or excited enthusiasm. However, we should keep in mind that those who condemn self-mutilation in the name of immoral vanity but, at the same time, accept mutilation in the name of religious traditions, falsely believe that the Devlinian "intolerance, indignation, and disgust" attitude provides sufficient grounds for constraining people's self-regarding behavior.

The general question is why would it be wrong to want to try to improve one's looks when people are usually encouraged to improve themselves in other respects? We are supposed to care for ourselves, keep ourselves fit, not offend others with bad personal hygiene and inappropriate clothing—not to mention that intellectual advancement has always been considered worthy of praise. Training of skills and cultivation of mental capacities are encouraged, sometimes at great expense: some emphasizing the intrinsic value of knowledge and some seeing education as instrumentally valuable. But is it only so because radical improvement of our physical appearance has so far been beyond our reach? Or is it perhaps so that even if beauty might be conducive to greater riches, the quest for it may get out of hand and become an obsession which could destroy us as easily as any other vice. After all, physical beauty—unlike beauty in art—is only a passing thing. As Dorian Gray's portraitist hears from his friend:

"Days in summer, Basil, are apt to linger," murmured Lord Henry. Perhaps you will tire sooner than he will. It is a sad thing to think of, but

there is no doubt that Genius lasts longer than Beauty. That accounts for
the fact that we all take such pains to over-educate ourselves. In the wild
struggle for existence, we want to have something that endures, and so
we fill our minds with rubbish and facts, in the silly hope of keeping our
place .... The mind of the thoroughly well-informed man is a dreadful
thing. It is like a bric-à-brac shop, all monsters and dust, with everything
priced above its proper value.[3]

4. Social Competition, Economic Pressure

So far, I have simply presumed that the demand for cosmetic surgery is just
another instance of autonomous choosing. But would it in fact be more
sensible to assume that behind this ever-increasing need is a strong social
pressure, pushing or even forcing both women and men towards these
operations. The desire for social and economic success creates competition and
tension which may present themselves both as a threat to lose one's job and as
a constant reminder to keep company's best interests in mind by taking good
care of one's looks. In such cases is it really possible to say that the person has
herself deemed it necessary to upgrade her looks? Or have we ended up with
the situation where the old traditions that once held us captive have simply
been replaced by new customs which we are to honor if we want to keep our
acquired status in the social stratum? As easily as the company can tell its
executives that it is not appropriate for someone in their position to ride a
bicycle to work (and of course insist on having them drive a Jaguar), they may
without any sense of guilt employ drastic measures in order to make people
realize how they are expected to look. And unfortunately it might be easier for
a male employee to stick to his bicycle—him being a known eccentric—than
for a female employee to stick to her old sagging face. We do have good
reason to ask whether all decisions to have major cosmetic surgery are taken
by individuals, who are adult, sane, aware of risk, calm and under no pressure.

One major ethical problem concerning the cosmetic business is related to
professional ethics. A doctor's duty has always been to try to alleviate pain and
suffering and if possible cure patients seeking their help. But in the case of
cosmetic surgeons the situation is different. The clinics advertising the latest
and finest operations are mainly interested in profit, and are trying to sell their
services whether the client really needs them or not. Or should we believe that
the doctors are eagerly trying to persuade their clients that their original nose
suits their face, or to convince them to forgo liposuction since a healthy diet
combined with physical exercise is just what they need?[4] This of course is
nothing unique since markets take care of our well-being in trying to sell us all
sorts of beautifying gimmicks, but it is fair to say that the difference between
the eager sales person behind the perfume counter and the plastic surgeon with
fancy diplomas is significant. The latter belongs to a class of highly respected

professionals who we believe to possess epistemic authority in medical matters. And many people may easily extend this authority to aesthetic assessments.

Responsible doctors with high moral integrity do not try to convince their patients that their lives will improve once they have subjected themselves to the scalpel. We wouldn't be too happy to hear about surgeons who try to convince their patients that in order to anticipate later troubles they should have their appendix operated or ophthalmologists who ridicule patients who prefer spectacles to laser operations. Why then are we ready to call physicians those business men whose main interest clearly lies in monetary profit? Do their well-advertised businesses fulfill the criteria of medical professionalism? At least in some cases, might it not be a good idea to start calling them cosmetic engineers instead of doctors?

It may be that one day our hubristic self-confidence and pride will destroy us in our endeavors to be young and immortal. But it seems to me that if it turns out to be a dream shared by many, we should not try to engage in a doomed fight against it. Most of us are rather moderate in our wish to feel youthful and will therefore be saved from Dorian Gray's regrets:

> It was his beauty that had ruined him, his beauty and the youth that he
> had prayed for. But for those two things, his life might have been free
> from stain. His beauty had been to him but a mask, his youth but a
> mockery. What was youth at best? A green, and unripe time, a time of
> shallow moods, and sickly thoughts. Why had he worn its livery? Youth
> had spoiled him.[5]

NOTES

1. Immanuel Kant, *Observations on the Feeling of the Beautiful and Sublime* [1763], translated by J. T. Goldthwait (Berkeley: University of California Press, 1960), p. 51.

2. *Ibid.*, p. 92.

3. Oscar Wilde, *The Picture of Dorian Gray* [1890] (Oxford: Oxford University Press, 1994), p. 12.

4. *Cf.* Carl Hiaasen, *Skin Tight* (New York: Pan Books, 1991).

5. Wilde, *The Picture of Dorian Gray*, p. 220.

Twenty-Three

NEW LIFE FORMS: MIN OR MAX CYBORGS?

Timo Airaksinen

1. Introduction

In this chapter I study two interesting versions of cyborg theory and cybersociety, presented by Andy Clark and Donna Haraway. The first one is technological, ontological, and minimalistic. The second is political, epistemological, and maximalistic. I introduce some methodological min and max concepts and speculate on reasoning inside-out, outside-in, top-down and bottom-up. Clark preaches the principles of cyborg construction but does not say much of what happens next. Haraway provides us with a picture of cyberworld without saying much of what its engineering features are. The obvious temptation to combine both approaches must be resisted, however. They are mutually incompatible. I try to indicate why this is so. I do not provide information about the details of Clark's and Haraway's thinking. In the end I speculate about new life forms, artificial life, artificial intelligence, and cyborgs. Clark as a social liberal technologist is a traditionalist thinker unlike Haraway whose radicalism goes deeper than one might think. It is not tied to any technological descriptions or predictions, and this is her great strength. This makes room for new life forms.

2. Two Views on Cyborg Metaphysics

A. Clark and Haraway

Donna Haraway sketches a maximalistic theory of cyborgs in her wonderfully prophetic "Cyborg Manifesto" (1985). Andy Clark creates his own minimal cyborgs according to his less prophetic but equally interesting *Natural-Born Cyborgs* (2003).
    Clark writes:

> New waves of almost invisible, user-sensitive, semi-intelligent, knowledge-based electronics and software are perfectly posed to merge seamlessly with individual biological brains. In so doing they will ultimately blur the boundary between the user and her knowledge-rich, responsive,

unconsciously operating electronic environments. More and more parts of our worlds will come to share the moral and psychological status of parts of our brains. We are already primed by nature to dovetail our minds to our worlds. Once the world starts dovetailing back in earnest, the last few seams must burst, and we will stand revealed: cyborgs without surgery, symbionts without sutures.

The conclusion above is as if it were borrowed from Haraway. She writes:

> Human beings, like any other component or subsystem, must be localized in a system architecture whose basic modes of operation are probabilistic, statistical. No objects, spaces or bodies are sacred in themselves; any component can be interfaced with any other if the proper standard, the proper code, can be constructed for processing signals in common language. Exchange in this world transcends the universal translation effected by capitalist markets that Marx analyzed so well. The privileged pathology affecting all kinds of components in this universe is stress—a communications breakdown.[1]

I shall try to show that Clark's and Haraway's ideas are mutually incompatible, although Clark may suggest the opposite. He wants after all to "annex wave upon wave of external elements and structures as part and parcel of their extended minds."

Haraway's approach is "outside-in" cybertheory, when Clark works "inside-out." These two approaches seem to exhaust the relevant alternatives and are mutually incompatible; therefore any cybertheorist and postmodern bioethicist should consider them carefully. Only two choices are available. One must choose, or forget this issue. It is not possible to write a less minimalistic theory of cyborgs than Clark's. According to him, cyborgs are made by adding technoparts and -systems to a human biocreature who grows into a cyborg. Paul Verhoeven's film *Robocop* (1987) is my favorite illustration. Intuitively this looks like the only possibility. The modern mind is procedurally technorational because it is natural to think in terms of machine construction: take a biobase and add functional technoparts to it and you get what you designed. If you need to know more about this process, you must enquire into the origins of the base and the new parts. Where do they come from? How are they made? Once you have done this, you know how the design was put together. You know what it is, just like an engineer does. And you know how it works.

Such an approach is inside-out because we start from a biocreature which we expand into something new by adding parts to him/her. The crucial question is this: What do we get if we continue this process of adding parts? Perhaps we get something radically new?

Haraway's approach differs from the technological engineering model, as sketched by Clark. She is a radical political thinker, in the sense that she assumes a cyberworld and its associated society and asks what has happened and how the new cyborgs are situated in it. She begins from what has happened, from a new cyberreality (outside) and then works toward the idea of the creatures who/which inhabit this novel world (inside). From the fact that it is a cyberworld, one can infer that it is inhabited by cyborgs. For her, the existence of a cyberworld is a sufficient condition of the existence of cyborgs.

B. The Key Terms

Let me explain the key terms:

Min cyborg: ontologically thinking, a minimally modified human being as a cyborg life form. Minimal technoparts (as implants) are sufficient to create such a cyborg. Unlike robots which are fully artificial cyborgs are technologically modified humans. If we add bioparts to robots, muscles for instance, we approach a cyborg from the opposite direction by creating a biologically modified robot. Can we start from a human being, add technoparts, and end up with a cyborg who/which is similar to a biorobot created by adding bioparts to a robot? I do not discuss the problem of whether cyborgs and biorobots can ever meet and mate. I find it strange, however, that the category of biorobots is discussed so seldom. *Max cyborg*: a cyborg which is modified so drastically that no "natural" human characteristics such as gender, race, or age apply anymore. Max approach says that cyborgs are "totally" different from natural human biocreatures. This is a political suggestion, as we will see. The difference between max and min cyborgs is a methodological one: min cyborgs are described in engineering terms by specifying what technoparts are added; max cyborgs are described as those technocreatures who fit in the new cyberworld. We need not know how they are built.

Next we need to focus on the application of the MiniMax method of evaluating the policies of change according to Clark. *MiniMax* is a method of evaluation of cyborg excellence. According to the MiniMax method we should minimize the maximal individual features of cyborgization which are seen as undesirable but necessary when we change a biocreature into a cyborg and an artificial life form. This is Clark's *inside-out* approach; you add to a human being artificial parts (inside) and this transforms him/her into something else which you then introduce to the social world (outside). You start from a natural human being and bring about an artificial creature, and you need not do much. It is enough to add minimal technoparts, such as a hearing aid connected directly and permanently to the auditive nerve. We can say that, to be successful, we minimize the technological changes and their effects on a human being. The greatest possible changes and effects are kept to the minimum so that between two equally functional cyborgs A and B, A is better if its techno-changes are smaller than B's. Such an approach is evolutionary. It is as if nothing has happened and yet it is a Brave New World. Clark seems to like it.

Haraway's radical method of evaluation is equally easy to understand. It means that maximal (revolutionary) techno-political alterations are accompanied by unspecified technologies. She wants to *maximize* social change in terms of the relevant postmodern parameters, like "sex/genetic engineering" and the "organism/biotic component"; she specifies 32 such pairs. The rule is: Max social effects with Min technological specifics. For instance, if cyber-reality does not recognize sex and gender, our old sexual parts are irrelevant, whether we still have them or not. Cyborgs have no gender or they have a variable gender regardless of whether they have sex organs or not. Genderlessness is a maximal social effect. This approach is still *outside-in* because here the social effects of technology are reflected in the characteristics of the individual creatures changing them in an unspecified manner, from natural to artificial and from bio to cyber things. The viewpoint is social-epistemological and not techno-ontological. The latter one tells us what technoparts are implanted in a human being to make him a cyborg, unlike the former which infers from social changes to individual (bio or techno) characteristics. In other words, the world has changed and so have humans. They are now cyborgs. The other approach focuses on the addition of technoparts and bypasses the problem of political effects.

C. Comparing the Two Systems

These two approaches are mutually incompatible and they exhaust the possibilities here. But is this so? First, consider the case against mutual compatibility. The following two theses show how things are:

> (i)   From the cyborg features of an artificial construction one cannot infer the politics of a cybersociety (Clark).
> (ii)   From the politics of a cybersociety we cannot infer the features of cyborgs (Haraway).

In order to unify Clark's and Haraway's approaches we need to refute the implications of (i) and (ii), but obviously we cannot do so. And if we keep both (i) and (ii), we cannot have a unified theory of cyborgs in a cybersociety. We need to choose one alternative as our starting point and forget the other one. In this sense (i) and (ii) are mutually incompatible.

The next issue is the case of completeness. Think about a minimal outside-in alternative. If I am right, this is impossible. What would it be like? Imagine first a society which is as close as possible to our current social reality, with most of its categories and distinctions intact, and then think of an individual cyborg induced by it. This approach seems to be totally uninteresting and ineffectual. Why speculate about a situation where nothing new is created? Social reality is as we know it and so are its individual members. Let us take an example. We already discussed the following case:

(a) Cybersociety no longer recognizes sex-based gender and that is why a cyborg's (bio) sex organs are irrelevant, even if they still exist.

The next case does not make sense. It is trivial:

(b) Cybersociety recognizes sex-based gender and that is why a cyborg's (bio) sex organs are relevant, if they still exist.

Alternative (b) is not worth stating. In (b) one can replace "cyborg" with "human" and nothing changes. We need to continue to list the human organs in order to find one whose function is lost or changed because of the cyberworld. But in (a) the same is not true. The sex organs are an essential part of a human being. If they are lost (in the social-epistemological sense), the human biobeing disappears too. Haraway's idea seems to be similar. Radical changes entail the loss of the human being. What replaces us?—cyborgs as techno beings. He/she becomes "it."

What can be said about a possible maximizing inside-out alternative? Is it equally uninteresting? It is, because first we need to create a cyberreality which is maximally different from our current social world and then fill it with technologically modified biocreatures or cyborgs. This procedure is either redundant or inconsistent. It contains too much information. It is redundant in the sense that in order to change our familiar modern society into postmodern cyberreality all we need to do is to introduce the relevant cybersystems technologies into it, according to Haraway's radical thesis. We do not need to consider the relevant individual modifications of biocreatures which make them cyborgs. They are already cyborgs. The suggested procedure is redundant because cyberreality as such implies the existence of cyborgs, yet now one proposes that humans be transformed into cyborgs. How can you do that, if no pure human biocreatures exist anymore? In other words, the maximal approach presupposed the existence of cyborgs, but to be viable the inside-out vision requires human biocreatures as starting points. This is conversationally inconsistent.

Jean Baudrillard writes: "the meticulous operation of technology serves as a model for the meticulous operation of the social ... this is the essence of socialization, which began centuries ago."[2] But we have already seen that such an engineering approach need not be the only game in town; on the contrary. Haraway shows that we can also write like this: the meticulous operation of the social serves as the model for the meticulous operation of the technological ... this is the essence of the technological. Inside-out is no privileged or "natural" perspective. Ontology is not everything. Outside-in is what "political" means in its epistemological sense. We know technology only as something social. If technology is not social, we have no use for it, as the school of Social Constructivism says about technology.[3] In other words, cyborgs are designed and built (Clark), but what they are is an epistemological and social question (Haraway). And these two approaches cannot be reduced to each other. They remain separate. For example: that some cyborgs are white and some are colored does not mean that a cybersociety recognizes color, race, and discrimination. Small cyborgs are not necessarily babies.

3. Evaluating New Life Forms

A. Traditional and Radical Cybersocieties

Cyborgs may constitute a new life form. Clark's minimal cyborgs hardly qualify as something new, which indicates a disappointing traditionalism. Technologically improved humans have been with us for a long time without creating overwhelming theoretical interest. Haraway does not say much about technology, as we have seen. But her construction is till closer to new life forms than Clark's. Actually Haraway's approach is at least open to radically novel interpretation, more so than Clark's which is tied to the mundane prospects of modern engineering. If he wants to say how new life forms are to be generated, he actually needs to make those inventions and innovations which are unknown to us now. He must tell us the story of how to engineer a cyborg which contains something which is so radically new, that we get the idea of a new life form. There is also one more constraint: no SciFi material is allowed. Of course there is no logical reason why Clark could not do it, but we can also say that there is no reason why he could do it.

   Haraway's case is much easier because she works outside-in. If she is able to describe a cybersociety and its politics so that her construction is novel and makes sense, she may have reached her goal. This is how I see it. Haraway wants to create a maximal cyborg outside-in. That is why she sketches a cybersocial order in her "Cyborg Manifesto." Suppose that society is completely networked so that members are connected to each other by means of a mobile interface permanently connected to one's central nervous system. Think of a mobile phone like a device plugged into one's brain stem and spinal cord. Everyone has it together with an ID chip under the skin and a GPS. Such a being is certainly a cyborg. However, we need not specify, as we did above, how the identification, localization, and connectivity of the cyborgs are achieved. Maximal effects (politically) may be achieved by means of minimal modifications. Networked, virtual, and collective consciousness and a life world mean a maximal change compared to the modern isolationistic life style. But at the same time individual cyborgs are minimally altered, and thus we need to know minimally about their techno changes. A couple of simple devices are enough. This is to say that they are cyborgs because of their social political world rather than their own physical modifications. The members of a cybersociety are cyborgs. This is the crucial idea. It is not the case that a cybersociety emerges because of cyborgs, however heavily modified they are. The same idea applies to the new life forms: in the new cybersociety we have them, regardless of the nature of the creatures which inhabit the new world. In the new society we are alive in a new sense of the old word.

B. Top-Down AI or Bottom-Up AL?

We can continue this story toward AI (artificial intelligence) and AL (artificial life). The first, AI, is traditionally associated with such ideas as the Turing test and top-down engineering.[4] The second, AL, means the bottom-up approach in an open ended and unpredictable evolutionary context.[5] Clark's minimal cyborgs are naturally AI oriented creatures whose intelligence may be more or less heavily technologically modified but it is still intelligence in the proper human sense of the word. He/she can pass the Turing test and negotiate his/her life and career in society. She may be superbly A-intelligent but her life is still lived in our traditional society where we classify people according to their IQ and rate their career prospects accordingly. Nothing has changed since the coming of the AI of cyborgs. The stupid are always among us.

Compare this with Haraway's maximal vision. In a cybersociety no division between the clever and stupid exists. We cannot talk about the different ways men and women think and emote. Perhaps even the distinction between rational thinking and irrational emoting is obsolete. What does this entail in terms of AI? Certainly it does not entail that all individual cyborgs are engineered and genetically modified to have a top IQ. Perhaps they do not have IQ at all? This is Haraway's radical point: We should not feel compelled to project our own tired social categories, such as intelligence, rationality and IQ on to the new reality of a cybersociety. It is a new world whose foundations are also new, a technological construct which is not directly connected to anything we used to know. It is populated by cyborgs who may well be AL based creatures, engineered bottom-up. They are evolving quickly, endlessly trying new ways and approaches, until they find an equilibrium. Next they go through a series of mutations again, creating something new. Fully networked and connected cyborgs with strong AL features become so fluid and ephemeral that they can hardly be called individual members of society anymore. They are flashes on an information network. In that sense they are truly maximal cyborgs who maximize the effects of their own technological features, whatever these are. The new cyborgs may well look just like we do now, but they are no longer living life as we know it. Clark's minimal cyborgs, however extensively modified, still live like us. They are modeled after us—what a pity!

NOTES

1. Andy Clark, *Natural Born Cyborgs* (Oxford: Oxford University Press, 2003), p. 34, and Donna Haraway, "A Cyborg Manifesto" (1985) in Neil Spiller, *Cyber Reader* (London: Phaidon, 2002), pp. 110-114, p. 111.

2. Jean Baudrillard, *Simulacra and Simulation* (Ann Arbor, MI: University of Michigan Press, 1994), p. 34.

3. W. E. Bijker, *Of Bicycles, Bakelites, and Bulbs: Toward a Theory of Sociotechnical Change* (Cambridge, MA: MIT Press, 1995).

4. John Searle, *Minds, Brains and Science* (Cambridge, MA: Harvard University Press, 1984).

5. Steven Johnson, *Emergence* (New York: Scribner, 2001); Eric Bonabeau, Marco Dorigo, and Guy Theraulaz, *Swarm Intelligence* (Oxford: Oxford University Press, 1999).

ABOUT THE AUTHORS AND EDITORS

TIMO AIRAKSINEN is Professor of Moral and Social Philosophy at the University of Helsinki, Finland. His research interests include philosophy of technology and Hobbes.

VILHJÁLMUR ÁRNASON studied philosophy at The University of Iceland (B.A.) and at Purdue University, USA (M.A., Ph.D). He was an Alexander von Humboldt scholar in Berlin (1993) and visiting fellow at Clare Hall Cambridge (2006). He is Professor of Philosophy and Chair of the Centre for Ethics at the University of Iceland. He works mainly in the fields of moral theory, bioethics and political philosophy.

RICHARD ASHCROFT is Professor of Bioethics in the School of Law, Queen Mary University of London, UK. He taught previously in the medical schools of Queen Mary, Imperial College London, and Bristol University. He is a Deputy Editor of the Journal of Medical Ethics. He works mainly in research ethics and public health ethics, but has a wide range of philosophical interests in applied ethics.

MARGARET PABST BATTIN is Distinguished Professor of Philosophy and Adjunct Professor of Internal Medicine in the Division of Medical Ethics and Humanities at the University of Utah, USA. The author of prize-winning short stories and recipient of the University of Utah's Distinguished Research Award, she has authored, edited, or co-edited nineteen books, including studies of philosophical issues in suicide, a volume of case-puzzles in aesthetics, a text on professional ethics, a study of ethical issues in organized religion, two collections of essays on end-of-life issues, entitled *The Least Worst Death* and *Ending Life*, and the multi-authored volumes *Drugs and Justice: Seeking a Consistent, Coherent, Comprehensive View* and *The Patient as Victim and Vector: Ethics and Infectious Disease*.

REBECCA BENNETT is Senior Lecturer in Bioethics, Centre for Social Ethics and Policy, and Institute for Science, Ethics and Innovation, University of Manchester, UK. Rebecca has published widely on diverse issues in bioethics since early 1990s. Her specific research interests include antenatal HIV testing, assisted reproductive technologies, preimplantation genetic diagnosis, genetic testing in pregnancy, arguments surrounding attempts to eradicate disability, responsibility in pregnancy, HIV/AIDS, cloning, stem cell research, ectogenesis, and selective treatment of infants.

LISA BORTOLOTTI is Senior Lecturer in Philosophy at the University of Birmingham, UK. Her main interests are in the philosophy of the cognitive sciences and in applied ethics. She has written articles on philosophical psychopathology for journals such as *Mind & Language*, *Phenomenology and the Cognitive Sciences*, and *Philosophical Psychology*. She has contributed to bioethical debates on reproductive autonomy and research ethics with articles in the *Journal of Medical Ethics*, *Reproductive Biomedicine Online*, *Theoretical Medicine and Bioethics*, and the *Cambridge Quarterly of Healthcare Ethics*. She is the author of *An Introduction to the Philosophy of Science* (Polity Press, 2008), the editor of *Philosophy and Happiness* (Palgrave Macmillan, 2009), and the co-editor with Matthew Broome of *Psychiatry as Cognitive Neuroscience: Philosophical Perspectives* (Oxford University Press, 2009).

TOM BULLER is Associate Professor of Philosophy at the University of Alaska Anchorage. His main research interests are in bioethics and neuroethics.

LESLIE P. FRANCIS is Distinguished Professor, Department of Philosophy, and Alfred C Emery Professor of Law at the University of Utah. She works on areas at the intersection of law, legal and ethical theory, bioethics, and disability. She is particularly interested in issues of distributive justice, partial compliance theory, and discrimination. She is co-editor of six volumes, including the *Blackwell Guide to Medical Ethics* and *Americans with Disabilities*, co-author of *Land Wars: Property, Community and Land Use in an Interconnected World*, and author of *Sexual Harassment: Ethical Issues in Academic Life*.

HETA GYLLING is Professor and Head of the Department of Social and Moral Philosophy at the University of Helsinki, Finland. Her fields of expertise include ethics and philosophy of law.

SVEN OVE HANSSON is Professor and Head of the Department of Philosophy and the History of Technology, Royal Institute of Technology, Stockholm, Sweden. He is editor-in-chief of *Theoria,* one of the directors of the Stockholm Centre for Healthcare Ethics, and board member of the international Society for Philosophy and Technology. He is the author of around 200 papers in international journals on a wide range of philosophical topics, including ethics, value theory, decision theory, philosophy of risk, philosophy of science and technology, epistemology, and formal logic. His books include *A Textbook of Belief Dynamics* (Kluwer 1999) and *The Structure of Values and Norms* (CUP 2001). Homepage: http://www.infra.kth.se/~soh.

JOHN HARRIS is Lord David Alliance Professor of Bioethics and Research Director in the Institute for Science, Ethics and Innovation at the University of Manchester, UK. He is a Fellow of the United Kingdom Academy of Medical Sciences and a member of the United Kingdom Human Genetics Commission. He holds a number of editorial positions including joint Editor-in-Chief of the *Journal of Medical Ethics*. John Harris is the author or editor of fifteen books and over two hundred papers.

MATTI HÄYRY is Professor of Bioethics and Philosophy of Law at the Centre for Social Ethics and Policy, University of Manchester, UK and Professorial Fellow at the Helsinki Collegium for Advanced studies, University of Helsinki, Finland. Matti is the author of 12 books including *Liberal Utilitarianism and Applied Ethics* (Routledge, 1994) and *Rationality and the Genetic Challenge* (Cambridge University Press, 2009). He holds a number of editorial positions and was the President of the International Association of Bioethics 2007-2009.

SIRKKU HELLSTEN is Adjunct Professor in Social and Moral Philosophy at the University of Helsinki, Finland. She has taught philosophy at the Universities of Helsinki, South Florida, USA, Birmingham, UK, and Dar-Es-Saleem, Tanzania. She currently works as Governance Counsellor at the Embassy of Finland in Nairobi, Kenya, continuing also her academic research and teaching activities.

PETER HERISSONE-KELLY is Lecturer in Philosophy in the International School for Communities, Rights, and Inclusion at the University of Central Lancashire, UK. He works mainly on the ethics of new reproductive technologies and on the theoretical foundations of bioethical inquiry.

SØREN HOLM is a cosmopolitan bioethicist. He was born and educated in Denmark but now lives in the UK and divides his academic life between the UK and Norway (and nice and sunny places where kind people invite him to attend workshops). He holds numerous academic degrees, two Chairs and a few editorships.

JAY A. JACOBSON is Professor of Internal Medicine, Emeritus Chief, Division of Medical Ethics and Humanities, and member, Division of Infectious Diseases, University of Utah School of Medicine and Intermountain Medical Center, USA. He is a Fellow of the American College of Physicians and member of its Ethics and Human Rights Committee; Fellow, Infectious Diseases Society of America; and Director, Utah Partnership to Improve End of Life Care. In 2004, he was given the American Medical Association Isaac

Hayes and John Bell Award for Leadership in Medical Ethics and Professionalism.

VEIKKO LAUNIS is Professor of Medical Ethics and Adjunct Professor of Ethics and Social Philosophy at the University of Turku, Finland.

HARRY LESSER was, until his retirement, a Senior Lecturer in Philosophy at Manchester University, and is now a part-time lecturer in Jurisprudence in the School of Law. He has published a number of articles in bioethics, and edited or co-edited three published collections of papers, in particular *Ageing, Autonomy and Resources* (Ashgate, 1999). He has recently completed editing a fourth collection, for Rodopi, entitled *Justice for Older People,* and two articles on the right to free movement of labor.

FRANK LEAVITT, whose friends call him by his Hebrew name, *Yeruham*, was with his wife, June, a homesteader in the forest of Western Massachusetts, an organic gardener and dairy goat raiser in Upstate New York, a mechanic for racing bicyclists, an irrigation worker and general repairman on a kibbutz in the Northern Sinai, a Hebron settler, an Israeli soldier, a glazier, and a plumber. He is also a philosophy graduate of John Carroll, Toronto and Edinburgh Universities and teaches since 1990 in the Faculty of Health Sciences, Ben Gurion University, Beer Sheva, Israel. Among his teaching subjects are biomedical ethics, philosophy of the health and life sciences, health in the Eastern and Western philosophy, and aging in Eastern and Western Philosophy.

PEKKA LOUHIALA is Lecturer in medical ethics at the University of Helsinki, Finland. He has degrees both in medicine and philosophy and he also works as a part-time pediatrician in private practice. He has published on various topics in medical ethics, philosophy of medicine and epistemology. His current academic interests include conceptual and philosophical aspects of issues like evidence based medicine, alternative medicine and placebo.

MICHAEL PARKER is Professor of Bioethics and Director of the Ethox Centre at the University of Oxford [www.ethox.org.uk], UK. His main research interest is in the ethical and social dimensions of collaborative global health research. He leads the ethics programme of the Malaria Genomic Epidemiology Network (MalariaGEN) [www.malariagen.net] which carries out genomic research into severe malaria in childhood at 24 sites in 21 countries (funded by the Wellcome Trust and the Bill and Melinda Gates Foundation through the Foundation for the National Institutes of Health as part of the Grand Challenges in Global Health initiative). He also leads the ethics programme of the MRC Centre for Genomics and Global Health and is the Principal Investigator of the Collaborative Global Health Research Ethics Network (funded by a Wellcome Trust Biomedical Ethics Enhancement Award). Michael's other research activities include: the use of medical records for research (funded by the Medical Research Council); ethics in cardiovascular genomics (funded by the European Commission); and the governance of genetic databases (funded by the Wellcome Trust).

JUHA RÄIKKÄ, PhD, teaches philosophy at the University of Turku, Finland. Räikkä was nominated as a docent at the University of Turku in 1994. He has worked as a researcher and a teacher since 1988, and as a professor at the department in Philosophy in Turku for seven years. In 2006 he was nominated as a Lecturer in Practical Philosophy. Räikkä is an editor of the Finnish philosophical journal *Ajatus*. Räikkä's research interests focus on ethics and political philosophy. He has published papers on issues such as global justice, population ethics, group rights, privacy, autonomy, guilt, self-deception, and conspiracy theory. Räikkä's recent publications include a book on Privacy (in Finnish: *Yksityisyyden filosofia*, WSOY, 2007), and he is the Co-Editor of *Genetic Democracy: Philosophical Perspectives* (Springer, 2008).

LARRY REIMER is Professor at the Department of Pathology, University of Utah, USA.

ROSAMOND RHODES, PhD, is Professor of Medical Education and Director of Bioethics Education at Mount Sinai School of Medicine, Professor of Philosophy at the Graduate Center, CUNY, and Professor of Bioethics and Associate Director of the Union-Mount Sinai Bioethics Program. She writes on a broad array of issues in bioethics. She is co-editor of *The Blackwell Guide to Medical Ethics* (Blackwell, 2007), *Medicine and Social Justice: Essays on the Distribution of Health Care* (Oxford, 2002), and *Physician Assisted Suicide: Expanding the Debate* (Routledge, 1998).

FLOORA RUOKONEN, PhD, is Science Adviser at the Academy of Finland. Her research interests include moral philosophy, the relationship of literature and philosophy, and philosophy of trust.

NIALL SCOTT is Senior Lecturer in Ethics in the International School for Communities, Rights and Inclusions at the University of Central Lancashire, UK. He has worked at UCLAN since 2004 when a certain Prof. Matti Häyry offered him a lectureship in the Centre for Professional Ethics. They have been chums ever since, except when Man City are playing Spurs. Niall's work covers a multitude of interests and he has published and researched in Bioethics and Political philosophy, Heavy Metal and Philosophy and has spoken internationally on these subjects. He is the course leader for the MA in Bioethics and

Medical Law at UCLAN and in addition to Bioethics teaches science fiction and philosophy, and film and philosophy. He is the co-author of *Altruism* (with Jonathan Seglow), secretary for the Association for Social and Legal philosophy (ALSP), a member of the ESPMH and the Anarchist Studies Network. Horns Up!

CHARLES B. SMITH, MD, is Emeritus Professor of Medicine at the University of Utah School of Medicine, USA. He previously served as Chief of the Division of Infectious Diseases at the University of Utah School of Medicine, and Associate Dean at the University of Washington School of Medicine. His research has focused on respiratory viral and bacterial infections, and in recent years particularly on ethical issues related to infectious diseases. He is co-editor of *Ethics and Infectious Disease.*

TUIJA TAKALA is Academy Research Fellow at the Academy of Finland and Adjunct Professor of Social and Moral Philosophy at the University of Helsinki, Finland. She is president-elect of the European Society for Philosophy of Medicine and Health Care and holds a number of international editorial positions. Her current research interests lie in the conceptual, methodological and theoretical aspects of philosophical bioethics.

LEILA TOIVIAINEN was born and educated in Finland but has lived overseas all of her adult life. She trained as a registered nurse and registered midwife at the Newcastle General, UK in the seventies and then emigrated first to New Zealand and then on to Australia, where she had a career in neonatal intensive care nursing. In the late eighties she started studying philosophy at the University of Tasmania where she obtained her doctorate in 2000. In the same year she became Adjunct Professor at the University of Helsinki, Finland. She has been teaching bioethics since 1994 and her main academic interest is in the philosophy of Nietzsche. Her hobbies are free-range chickens, yoga and surfing.

SIMO VEHMAS is Professor of Special Education at the University of Jyväskylä, Finland. He is specialized in philosophical issues related to disability.

PAOLO VINEIS is Professor and Chair of Environmental Epidemiology at Imperial College London, UK, and Adjunct Professor of Epidemiology at Columbia University, New York, USA. His main field of work is cancer epidemiology, and in particular: (a) environmental causes of cancer; (b) the use of laboratory methods applied to the study of cancer etiology in populations; and (c) gene-environment interactions. Since 1992 he has coordinated the Turin section of the large EPIC study, a prospective study on diet and cancer. He is a member of the Steering Committee of EPIC and currently PI in projects on:

biomarkers, environmental exposures and cancer; genome-wide association studies on hypertension; air pollution and total mortality in Europe; and a European database on biomarkers for molecular epidemiology (ECNIS). Main methodological contributions have been in the evaluation of interactions of environmental and genetic risk factors; the concepts of causality in epidemiology; the integration and validation of –omics in epidemiology. Main didactic contributions have been in the organization of several editions of a Course of Molecular Epidemiology in collaboration with IARC (Lyon), the Leeds University and the Columbia University, New York. He is Course Director, BSc course on Global and Environmental Health at Imperial College. He has about 400 publications in PubMed, plus several books and chapters in books, e.g. *The Molecular Epidemiology of Chronic Diseases* (edited with Wild and Garte, Wiley Press, 2008).

SIMON WOODS is Senior Lecturer at the Policy, Ethics and Life Sciences Research Centre (PEALS), University of Newcastle, UK where he is the Director of Learning. PEALS is an ethics "Think Tank" involved in research teaching and public engagement on the ethical and social implications of the life sciences. Simon spent 10 years as a clinical cancer nurse and holds bachelor and doctoral degrees in philosophy. He has conducted empirical and conceptual research in bioethics. His current research concerns the ethical and social implications of early human development research, medical nanotechnology, and translational research in neuromuscular diseases.

INDEX

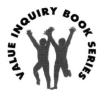

VIBS

The **Value Inquiry Book Series** is co-sponsored by:

Titles Published

187. Michael Krausz, *Interpretation and Transformation: Explorations in Art and the Self*. A volume in **Interpretation and Translation**

188. Gail M. Presbey, Editor, *Philosophical Perspectives on the "War on Terrorism."* A volume in **Philosophy of Peace**

189. María Luisa Femenías, Amy A. Oliver, Editors, *Feminist Philosophy in Latin America and Spain*. A volume in **Philosophy in Latin America**

190. Oscar Vilarroya and Francesc Forn I Argimon, Editors, *Social Brain Matters: Stances on the Neurobiology of Social Cognition*. A volume in **Cognitive Science**

191. Eugenio Garin, *History of Italian Philosophy*. Translated from Italian and Edited by Giorgio Pinton. A volume in **Values in Italian Philosophy**

192. Michael Taylor, Helmut Schreier, and Paulo Ghiraldelli, Jr., Editors, *Pragmatism, Education, and Children: International Philosophical Perspectives*. A volume in **Pragmatism and Values**

193. Brendan Sweetman, *The Vision of Gabriel Marcel: Epistemology, Human Person, the Transcendent*. A volume in **Philosophy and Religion**

194. Danielle Poe and Eddy Souffrant, Editors, *Parceling the Globe: Philosophical Explorations in Globalization, Global Behavior, and Peace*. A volume in **Philosophy of Peace**

195. Josef Šmajs, *Evolutionary Ontology: Reclaiming the Value of Nature by Transforming Culture*. A volume in **Central-European Value Studies**

196. Giuseppe Vicari, *Beyond Conceptual Dualism: Ontology of Consciousness, Mental Causation, and Holism in John R. Searle's Philosophy of Mind*. A volume in **Cognitive Science**

197. Avi Sagi, *Tradition vs. Traditionalism: Contemporary Perspectives in Jewish Thought*. Translated from Hebrew by Batya Stein. A volume in **Philosophy and Religion**

198. Randall E. Osborne and Paul Kriese, Editors, *Global Community: Global Security*. A volume in **Studies in Jurisprudence**